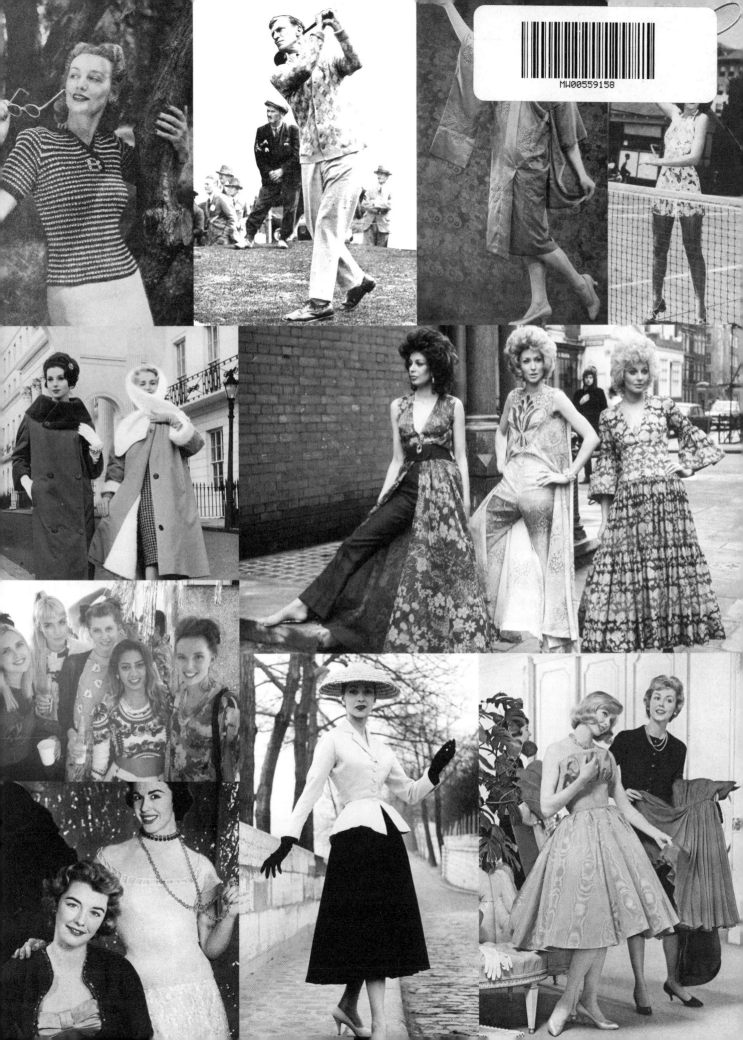

Happy
Birthday
Stephanie

— Love Lien 2017

THE VINTAGE FASHION BIBLE

WAYNE &
GERARDINE
HEMINGWAY

THE VINTAGE FASHION BIBLE

WAYNE &
GERARDINE
HEMINGWAY

THE STYLE GUIDE TO VINTAGE LOOKS
1920s – 1990s

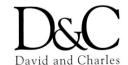
D&C
David and Charles

Contents

Introductiom   6

1920s   14
Women's day wear   16
Men's day wear   18
Women's evening wear   20
Men's evening wear   22
Shoes   24
Sportswear   26
Accessories   28
Get the Look with Hannah   30

Ask the Expert: Hats   32

1930s   34
Women's day wear   36
Men's day wear   38
Women's evening wear   40
Men's evening wear   42
Shoes   44
Sportswear   46
Accessories   48
Get the Look with Hannah   50

Ask the Expert: Buttons   52

1940s   54
Women's day wear   56
Men's day wear   60
Women's evening wear   64
Men's evening wear   68
Shoes   70
Sportswear   72
Accessories   74
Get the Look with Hannah   76

1950s   78
Women's day wear   80
Men's day wear   84
Women's evening wear   88
Men's evening wear   92
Shoes   94
Sportswear   96
Accessories   98
Get the Look with Hannah   100

Vintage Weddings   102

1960s 112
Women's day wear 114
Men's day wear 118
Women's evening wear 122
Shoes 124
Sportswear 126
Accessories 128
Get the Look with Hannah 130

Ask the Expert: Make-Up 132

1970s 134
Women's day wear 136
Men's day wear 142
Women's evening wear 146
Men's evening wear 150
Shoes 152
Sportswear 154
Accessories 156
Get the Look with Hannah 158

1980s 160
Women's day wear 162
T-shirts 166
Men's day wear 168
Women's evening wear 172

Men's evening wear 174
Shoes 176
Sportswear 178
Accessories 180
Get the Look with Hannah 182

1990s 184
Men & women's wear 186
Get the Look with Hannah 192
Future vintage 194

Buying Vintage 196

**Ask the Expert:
 Collecting Vintage** 200

Directory 202

Caring & Repairing 206

Glossary 214
About the Authors 218
Contributors 218
Picture credits 220
Index 221

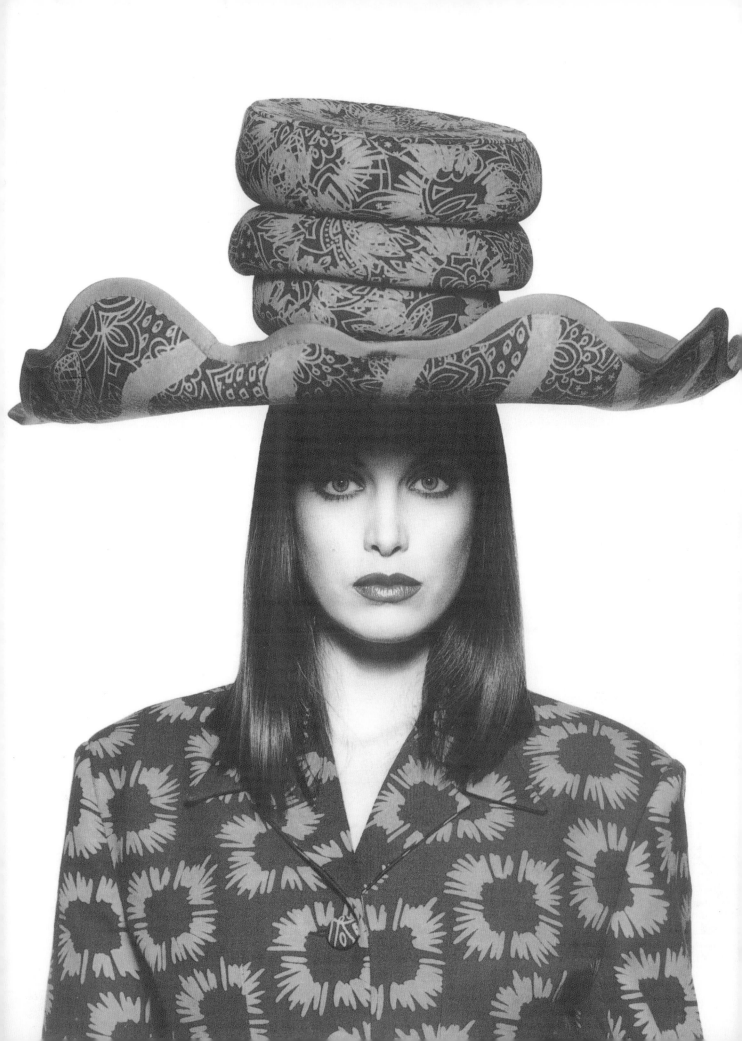

Introduction

As we steam ahead in the twenty-first century, anyone with their fashion head screwed on correctly will have some vintage stuff in their wardrobe. Not so long ago, wearing second-hand clothes was judged as a badge of poverty; however the clever and fortuitous rebranding of the market for classic, pre-worn clothes as 'vintage' has brought about a change in public perception and attitude. Now, quite rightly, collecting and/or wearing vintage is seen as both cool and creative, and the taste for vintage means it can be seen everywhere around the world, from the high street to the red carpet. Most excitingly, this change embraces sustainability; we should (I would like to say must) all preserve and celebrate good design and craftsmanship. Choosing to wear vintage (even if you own only one or two items) is not only about living sensibly, but there is also magic in the relationship. There will always be a certain intriguing satisfaction to be gained from owning and wearing a piece of clothing that already has a life story…and giving it another.

People often ask me, 'What is vintage?'

It is hard to find a source anywhere that gives a sensible answer or one that is easy to apply. So the time is ripe to set the parameters. In my view, an item of clothing's vintage tag can only be valid if it is a classic piece of design that has stood the test of time. And it is pretty much impossible to judge whether it has done that if it is less than 20 years old; a three-year-old dress from Topshop is most definitely not vintage!

My wife Gerardine and I have spent our lives steeped in timeless design, thrift and upcycling. The three combine to be our lifestyle choice and our design aesthetic. But, flicking through the titles on this subject matter, it became very clear to me that a book was needed that could

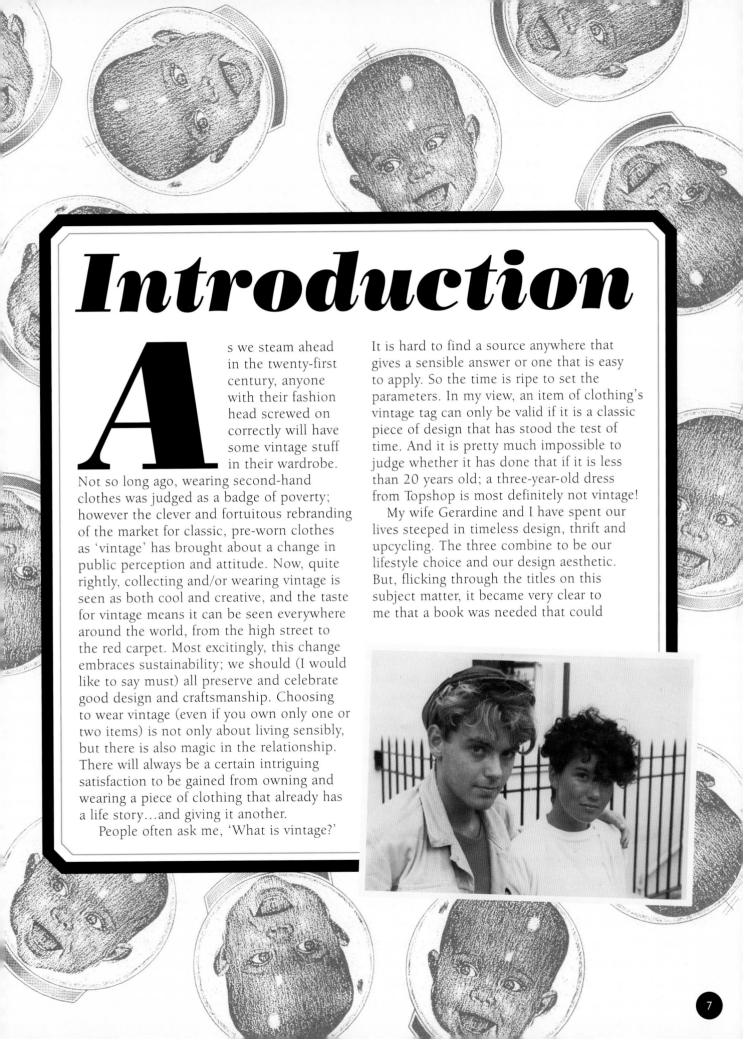

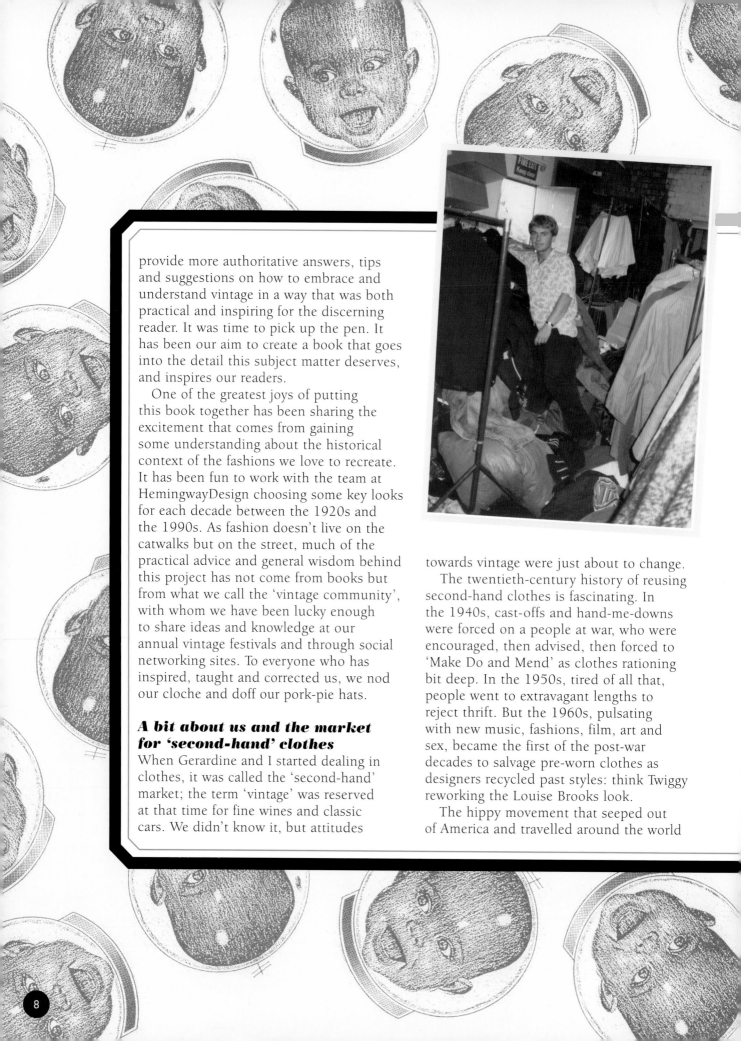

provide more authoritative answers, tips and suggestions on how to embrace and understand vintage in a way that was both practical and inspiring for the discerning reader. It was time to pick up the pen. It has been our aim to create a book that goes into the detail this subject matter deserves, and inspires our readers.

One of the greatest joys of putting this book together has been sharing the excitement that comes from gaining some understanding about the historical context of the fashions we love to recreate. It has been fun to work with the team at HemingwayDesign choosing some key looks for each decade between the 1920s and the 1990s. As fashion doesn't live on the catwalks but on the street, much of the practical advice and general wisdom behind this project has not come from books but from what we call the 'vintage community', with whom we have been lucky enough to share ideas and knowledge at our annual vintage festivals and through social networking sites. To everyone who has inspired, taught and corrected us, we nod our cloche and doff our pork-pie hats.

A bit about us and the market for 'second-hand' clothes

When Gerardine and I started dealing in clothes, it was called the 'second-hand' market; the term 'vintage' was reserved at that time for fine wines and classic cars. We didn't know it, but attitudes towards vintage were just about to change.

The twentieth-century history of reusing second-hand clothes is fascinating. In the 1940s, cast-offs and hand-me-downs were forced on a people at war, who were encouraged, then advised, then forced to 'Make Do and Mend' as clothes rationing bit deep. In the 1950s, tired of all that, people went to extravagant lengths to reject thrift. But the 1960s, pulsating with new music, fashions, film, art and sex, became the first of the post-war decades to salvage pre-worn clothes as designers recycled past styles: think Twiggy reworking the Louise Brooks look.

The hippy movement that seeped out of America and travelled around the world

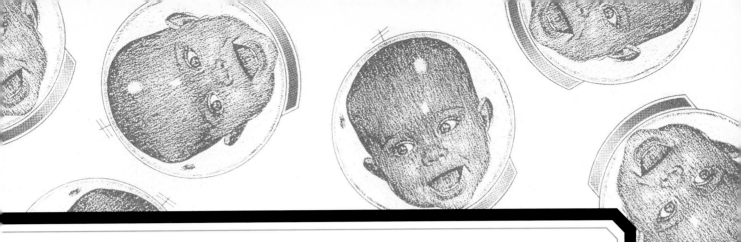

rejected new clothing and mass-produced synthetic materials as it renounced the ideals of capitalism and consumerism. The peace-movement protesters raided army-surplus stores in an ironic channelling of the military look. And in searching out used jeans to customize, old fur jackets to team with crêpe dresses and antique lace petticoats, the hippies reinvigorated the old flea markets, junk shops and newly established charity shops. As with all fashions, this look soon spread onto the street to the places where the young met, and in time it fed into the glam rock movement, and then punk, both of which looked to pre-worn clothes as a source for individual expression. And yet, up until the beginning of the 1980s, second-hand was still perceived in most circles as dirty and unhygenic and only for those who were not very well off. Wearing second-hand clothes at that time was a bold underground statement, a nightclub thing and a strong anti-establishment thing.

Me as a boy

I grew up in the seaside town of Morecambe in the north of England in the 1960s, in a household surrounded by fashion, music and thrift. Morecambe had few boutiques and my Mum and my Nan made most of their own clothes, taking inspiration from magazines and using the *Vogue* patterns scattered around the house – as were the albums of the Beatles and the Rolling Stones.

My mother was into glam rock and when I was ten she took me to see the band Sweet in concert. It was the start of a lifelong music addiction; it was exciting, but it wasn't just about the music, it was about clothes, too. By the age of 12, I had seen David Bowie's *Aladdin Sane* tour and I had decided to be different. Using my Nan's perforated swim cap, I bleached blonde highlights into my hair – getting into real trouble at school – and realized that while I couldn't afford to buy fashionable clothes, picking out the right second-hand garment opened up possibilities for individuality. I worked out where to find 1950s brothel creepers to mix with forties and fifties army-surplus gear to team with contemporary 1970s psychedelic T-shirts.

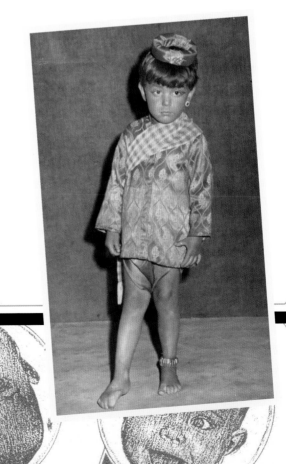

An obsession with clubbing soon followed, and my life began to revolve around the northern soul clubs and New York-style discos that proliferated in Lancashire towns of the north west. Then, when I was 15, punk broke out. The Sex Pistols played one of their first gigs in Blackburn at Lodestar and I was hooked. On their trail, I went down to London and beat a path to Vivienne Westwood's shop, *Seditionaries*, at World's End in Chelsea. T-shirts here were £80, whereas the train fare had only been about £8 (and a gig probably no more than £2), so I copied the look with second-hand clothes. I upcycled army fatigues into bondage trousers and ripped up a 1960s T-shirt, turning it into punk fashion. Back home, mid-week we went to punk clubs; weekends were northern soul and disco. It was often the same crowd at both, but we dressed differently depending on which scene we were in. For me, the disco look was influenced greatly by August Darnell (who performed as Kid Creole) and we scoured print magazines like *Blues&Soul* and *Black Music* to see what was happening in New York, where we discovered that Studio 54 was flirting with forties and fifties glamour. At about this time, the late 1970s, discerning second-hand clothes dealers started up here and there, but though we may have idolized Bryan Ferry, we couldn't afford to dress like him, even from these new, very cool shops. Instead, we sought

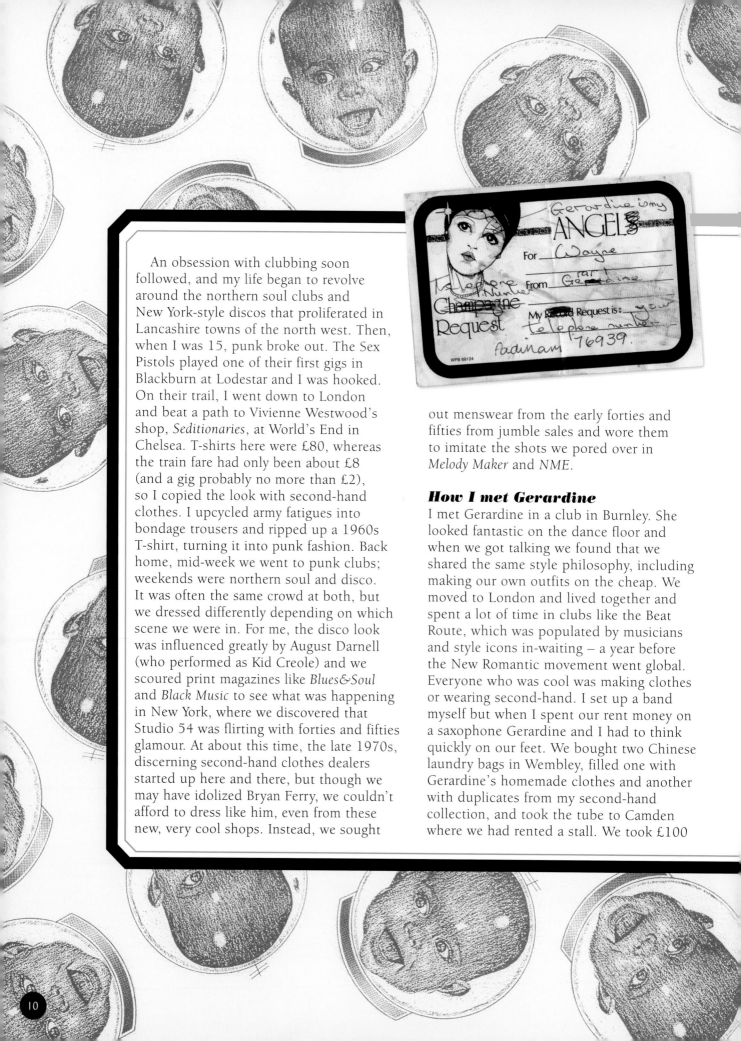

out menswear from the early forties and fifties from jumble sales and wore them to imitate the shots we pored over in *Melody Maker* and *NME*.

How I met Gerardine

I met Gerardine in a club in Burnley. She looked fantastic on the dance floor and when we got talking we found that we shared the same style philosophy, including making our own outfits on the cheap. We moved to London and lived together and spent a lot of time in clubs like the Beat Route, which was populated by musicians and style icons in-waiting – a year before the New Romantic movement went global. Everyone who was cool was making clothes or wearing second-hand. I set up a band myself but when I spent our rent money on a saxophone Gerardine and I had to think quickly on our feet. We bought two Chinese laundry bags in Wembley, filled one with Gerardine's homemade clothes and another with duplicates from my second-hand collection, and took the tube to Camden where we had rented a stall. We took £100

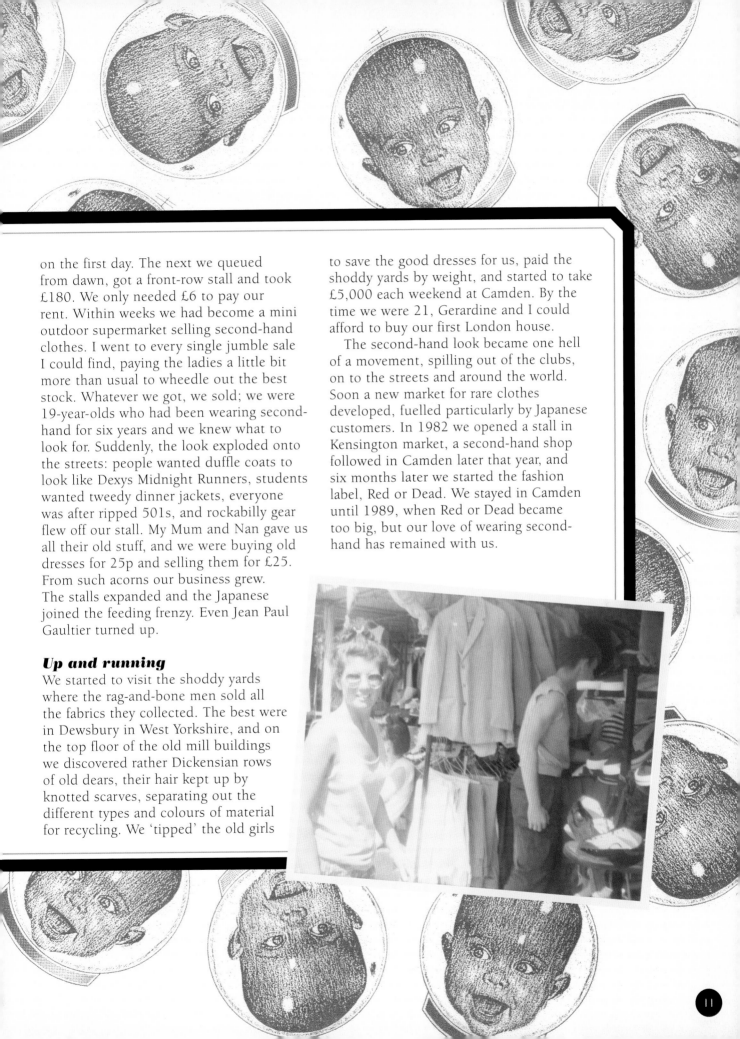

on the first day. The next we queued from dawn, got a front-row stall and took £180. We only needed £6 to pay our rent. Within weeks we had become a mini outdoor supermarket selling second-hand clothes. I went to every single jumble sale I could find, paying the ladies a little bit more than usual to wheedle out the best stock. Whatever we got, we sold; we were 19-year-olds who had been wearing second-hand for six years and we knew what to look for. Suddenly, the look exploded onto the streets: people wanted duffle coats to look like Dexys Midnight Runners, students wanted tweedy dinner jackets, everyone was after ripped 501s, and rockabilly gear flew off our stall. My Mum and Nan gave us all their old stuff, and we were buying old dresses for 25p and selling them for £25. From such acorns our business grew. The stalls expanded and the Japanese joined the feeding frenzy. Even Jean Paul Gaultier turned up.

Up and running

We started to visit the shoddy yards where the rag-and-bone men sold all the fabrics they collected. The best were in Dewsbury in West Yorkshire, and on the top floor of the old mill buildings we discovered rather Dickensian rows of old dears, their hair kept up by knotted scarves, separating out the different types and colours of material for recycling. We 'tipped' the old girls

to save the good dresses for us, paid the shoddy yards by weight, and started to take £5,000 each weekend at Camden. By the time we were 21, Gerardine and I could afford to buy our first London house.

The second-hand look became one hell of a movement, spilling out of the clubs, on to the streets and around the world. Soon a new market for rare clothes developed, fuelled particularly by Japanese customers. In 1982 we opened a stall in Kensington market, a second-hand shop followed in Camden later that year, and six months later we started the fashion label, Red or Dead. We stayed in Camden until 1989, when Red or Dead became too big, but our love of wearing second-hand has remained with us.

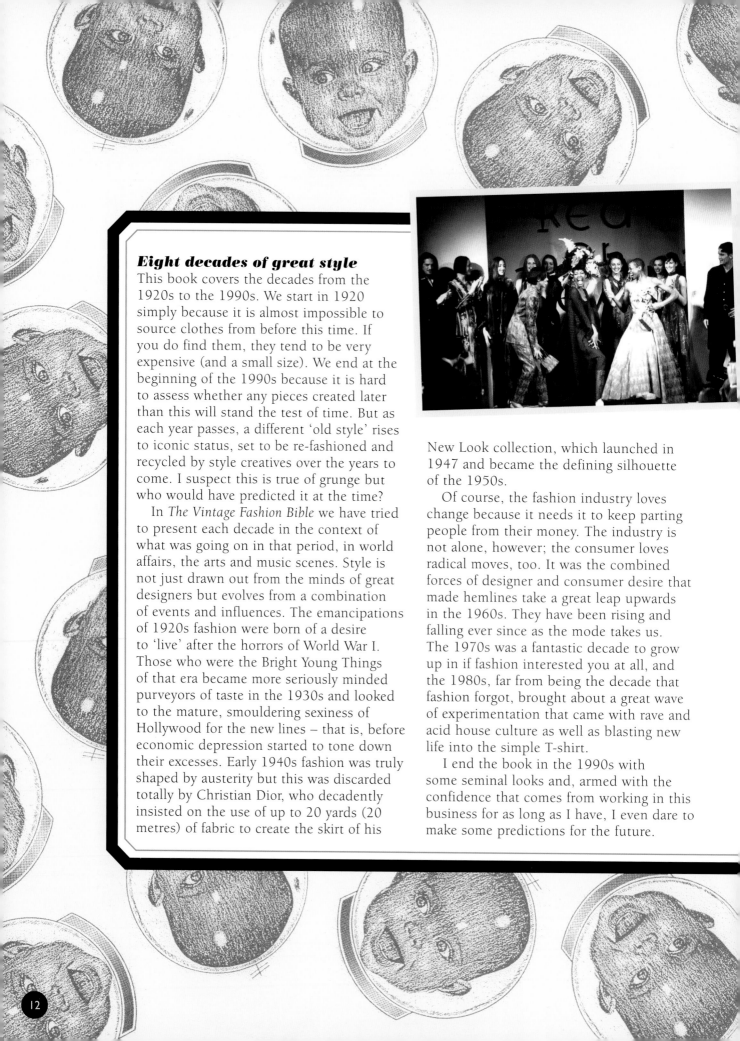

Eight decades of great style

This book covers the decades from the 1920s to the 1990s. We start in 1920 simply because it is almost impossible to source clothes from before this time. If you do find them, they tend to be very expensive (and a small size). We end at the beginning of the 1990s because it is hard to assess whether any pieces created later than this will stand the test of time. But as each year passes, a different 'old style' rises to iconic status, set to be re-fashioned and recycled by style creatives over the years to come. I suspect this is true of grunge but who would have predicted it at the time?

In *The Vintage Fashion Bible* we have tried to present each decade in the context of what was going on in that period, in world affairs, the arts and music scenes. Style is not just drawn out from the minds of great designers but evolves from a combination of events and influences. The emancipations of 1920s fashion were born of a desire to 'live' after the horrors of World War I. Those who were the Bright Young Things of that era became more seriously minded purveyors of taste in the 1930s and looked to the mature, smouldering sexiness of Hollywood for the new lines – that is, before economic depression started to tone down their excesses. Early 1940s fashion was truly shaped by austerity but this was discarded totally by Christian Dior, who decadently insisted on the use of up to 20 yards (20 metres) of fabric to create the skirt of his

New Look collection, which launched in 1947 and became the defining silhouette of the 1950s.

Of course, the fashion industry loves change because it needs it to keep parting people from their money. The industry is not alone, however; the consumer loves radical moves, too. It was the combined forces of designer and consumer desire that made hemlines take a great leap upwards in the 1960s. They have been rising and falling ever since as the mode takes us. The 1970s was a fantastic decade to grow up in if fashion interested you at all, and the 1980s, far from being the decade that fashion forgot, brought about a great wave of experimentation that came with rave and acid house culture as well as blasting new life into the simple T-shirt.

I end the book in the 1990s with some seminal looks and, armed with the confidence that comes from working in this business for as long as I have, I even dare to make some predictions for the future.

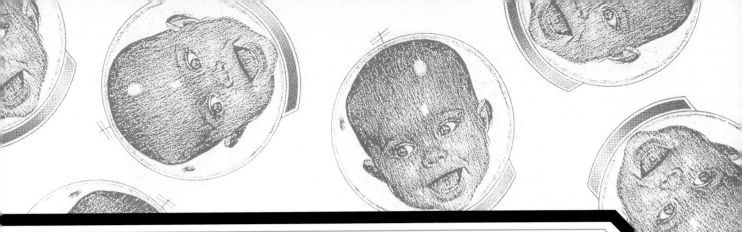

A note on sourcing

There are many places to find second-hand clothes, and it is also possible to source some gorgeous and beautifully made classic old pieces without going to a specialist dealer, but you need to keep your eyes open. The satisfaction of finding the perfect item in your size is incomparable and, from the right place, won't break the bank. In early 2013 I bought a handmade checked jacket for about $50 from the Williamsburg market in New York. Very similar, and not so well made, jackets were being sold in a popular globally branded upmarket store for five times that price.

An aside on underpinning and sizing

With vintage clothes you have more options if you are small-bodied. This is not a sizest comment favouring the stick-thin models that steal the limelight these days; I say this only because our forebears were smaller. As a result, old sizing labels bear no resemblance to those of the present day, just as old shoes were made to fit smaller, narrower feet. Gerardine and I, being a tad on the short side and pretty slim, have a big advantage in that we fit most all forties, fifties and sixties clothes.

When buying, use your common sense and try things on. But don't forget that with better diet and changes in lifestyle, body shapes have changed, as has the underwear designed to 'mould' the body to fit the fashion. The hourglass figures of the 1950s were not created by nature alone – corsetry and foundation garments helped.

A footnote on upcycling

Upcycling is the process of taking something that has seen better days and giving it new life. It is about being resourceful and grateful. It is great if you can do it yourself but not everyone is handy with a needle or has the kind of eye that can see all the possibilities. In buying upcycled fashion from other people you are sustaining an industry that repurposes goods, and that is a great thing to do.

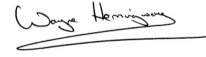

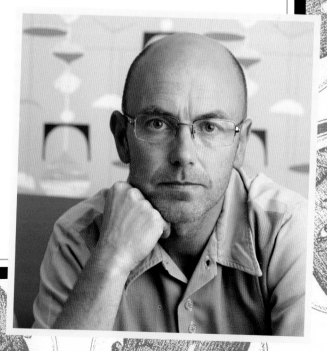

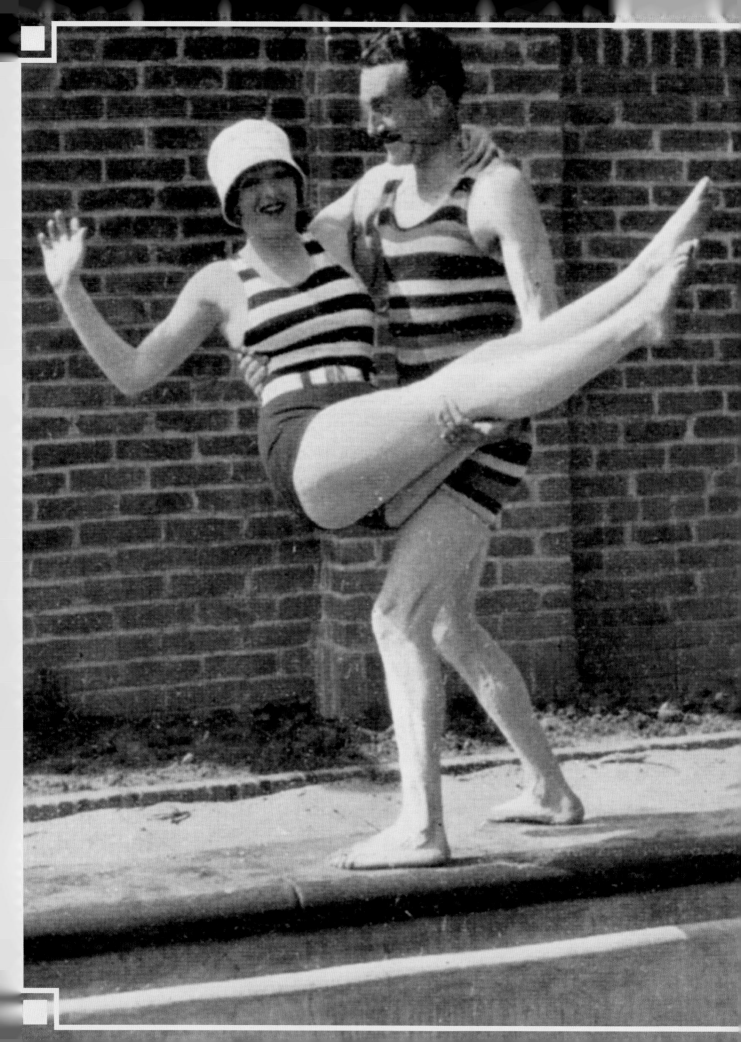

After the horrors of World War I most people were determined to live life to the full. The new decade brought an optimism and energy that was apparent in all areas of fashion. This was a period that broke all the rules in women's fashion, but the twenties weren't only about 'her' look. Attitudes and styles were also relaxing in men's tailoring, and there was an acceptance of a more casual way of dressing, which still influences styles today.

The excitement of this glorious, rebellious time was best demonstrated by the clothes of the 'Bright Young Things'. Girls cut their hair short and found the perfect accessory in the cloche hat. Dancing had never been so popular, and dresses, skirts and tunics were cut to allow freedom of movement. Beading and fringing were all the rage, and ankles, legs and backs were revealed. As the decade progressed, waistlines dropped and hemlines rose, shocking the world with a view of women's legs for the first time. But it was the rejection of corsets and the pursuit of the straight silhouette that dominated the decade. Overt femininity was slowly repressed in favour of a boyish silhouette, which was labelled the *garçonne* (little boy). Coco Chanel championed the look, which created shock and awe amongst traditionalists and paved the way for a more androgynous fashion trend that we take for granted in modern society.

Advances in fabric technology and dyes meant that 'luxury' materials, such as silk, could be imitated; the development of rayon resulted in brighter, cheaper fabrics being available for those of more modest means. Also, the burgeoning catalogue market, and a greater availability of sewing patterns, allowed fashionable styles to flow down from the higher echelons of the ateliers in Paris and London to the general public. But after such an optimistic and energetic start the 1920s ended with the stockmarket crash on Wall Street and the Great Depression on both sides of the Atlantic.

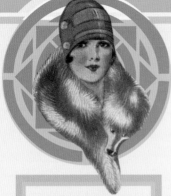

DESIGNERS

In the years following World War I, there was a notable increase in magazine articles about fashion. The designer you favoured and where you bought your outfits were hot topics. The wardrobe choices of high-profile personalities were increasingly influenced by fashion 'experts', who would comment on what was the 'must have' look of the season. This brought about fierce competition in high society as women began competing to employ the skills of in-demand designers, such as Coco Chanel, seen below in one of her own designs.

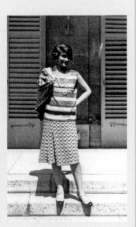

In the 1920s there was one word that was used more than any other: 'flapper'. The term was originally used in the UK to describe a young prostitute. However, during the 1920s it was used to describe the rebellious, high-spirited young women of the day who drank, smoked, danced and were determined to have fun. A typical flapper dress was straight cut with spaghetti straps – a style best suited to slim young women with a small bust and hips. All curves were completely abandoned and, with the new short hairstyles, heroines of popular novels were often described as being 'boyish'. The essence of fashion in this period revolved around freedom and the liberation from stiffness. The huge increase in the popularity of dancing, especially to jazz music, meant that styles became less complicated and more practical. Necklines remained round or 'V-shaped', and dresses were often styled by sewn-in belts, as designers concentrated on how the fabric moved with, and draped upon, the body.

Detailing was important, so tying, buttoning and layering were echoed in both high street and haute couture. Fashion and the arts became obsessed by exoticism and the Orient following the discovery in Egypt in 1922 of Tutankhamen's tomb and all the wonderful things it contained.

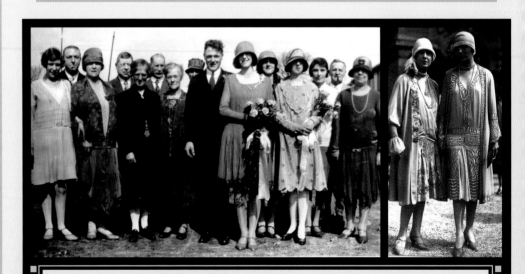

Photography had yet to supersede fashion illustration in the twenties. However, portraits and family photographs capture period style in all its glory. The wedding photo (above) shows guests wearing dresses with dropped waists, and scalloped and pointed hemlines. The lady on the far right has a godet in her dress skirt with kick pleats, reflecting the latest fashion trends.

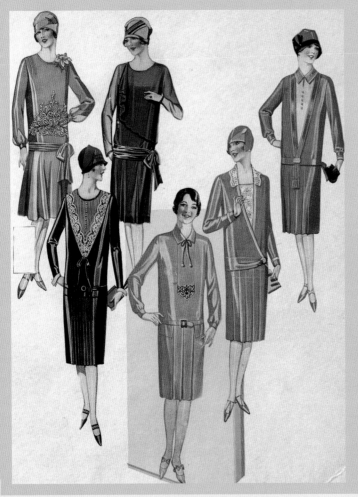

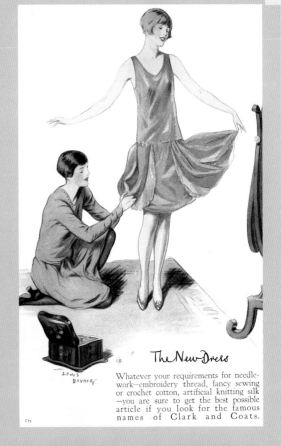

The New Dress

Whatever your requirements for needle-work—embroidery thread, fancy sewing or crochet cotton, artificial knitting silk —you are sure to get the best possible article if you look for the famous names of Clark and Coats.

BEE'S KNEES

Hems and waistlines dictated 1920s fashion. In 1923, waistlines fell somewhere between the natural waist and the hips, and by 1924 had progressed entirely to the hips. By the early part of 1926, the flapper dress had taken its most popular form with the waist in line with the lower hip and upper thigh.

Hemlines, previously referred to as skirt lengths, were typically just above the ankle or mid shin at the turn of the decade. They fell again in 1923, gradually rising back up from 1924 to somewhat shockingly expose the knee by 1927. At this point hemlines started to descend again, largely due to controversy and public concern about the morality of young women and the distracting effect short hemlines might have on men.

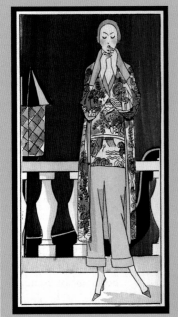

TROUSERS

Designers such as Schiaparelli and Chanel, courted controversy when they started to champion leisure trousers for ladies. Their designs were for high-waist, wide-leg trousers that finished at the ankle. Worn with long, loose tunic tops and teamed with oversize straight-cut blazers, all were made from lightweight fabrics. This sophisticated look was often completed with a close-fitting hat or headscarf and flat, strappy sandals, making it the perfect attire for holidays and informal events in warm weather.

The bar was set for many future 'classics' in an era in which just about every man, whatever his class or wealth, strove to look smart. Even factory workers went to work in a suit and hat, with those of more limited means still owning a separate suit for 'Sunday best'. Affluent gentlemen, of course, had a suit and hat for every occasion and pairs of plus fours for country pursuits. In many ways, men of the 1920s still dressed very much as their fathers had before them, at a time when no one would leave the house without a hat or a cap. Suits were generally made from heavy cloth, accompanied by a waistcoat, and the dapper gent would ensure a handkerchief was tucked into his breast pocket with the other pocket free for his fob watch.

For the younger generation formality was waning in many ways. Suit jackets were designed to be slim fitting, with shoulders and sleeves that hugged the body, in a style that pervaded the entire decade. Trousers retained a high waist and some were styled with wide legs and often up to a 58 cm (23-inch) circumference at the hem – referred to as Oxford Bags. In the 1920s, London usurped Paris as the hub of men's tailoring, particularly with England's reputation for excellent wool manufacture and the popularity of some members of the Royal Family who were revered for their fashion sense.

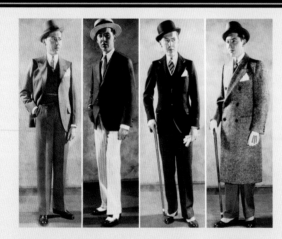

MATERIAL GUY

Wool, wool tweed and wool-based flannel were the preferred choice for suit material in the twenties. The fit was all important as suits were mainly made-to-measure. Style dictated acceptance of either single- or double-breasted jackets with either three or four buttons. The top button would sit on the left, over the heart, with the decade's signature notch lapels and double flap pockets. Matching trousers had a sharp centre crease and began to have turn-ups early into the decade. This trend continued throughout the period and well into the thirties.

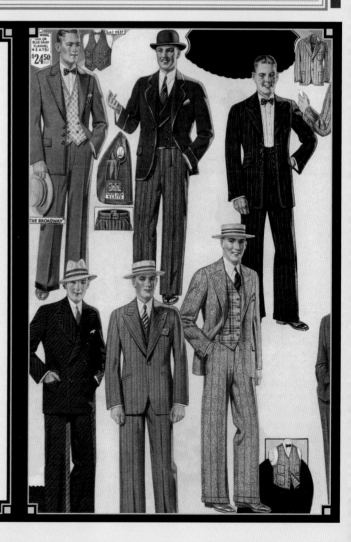

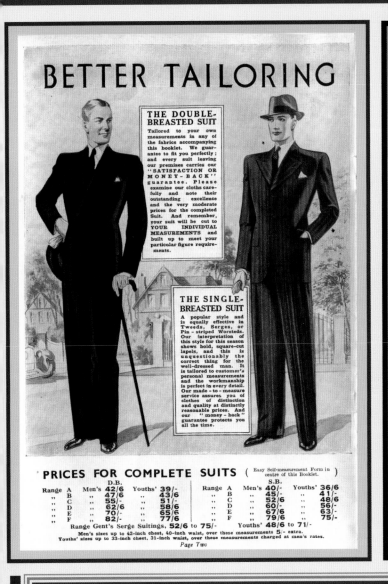

BETTER TAILORING

THE DOUBLE-BREASTED SUIT

Tailored to your own measurements in any of the fabrics accompanying this booklet. We guarantee to fit you perfectly; and every suit leaving our premises carries our "SATISFACTION OR MONEY-BACK" guarantee. Please examine our cloths carefully and note their outstanding excellence and the very moderate prices for the completed Suit. And remember, your suit will be cut to YOUR INDIVIDUAL MEASUREMENTS and built up to meet your particular figure requirements.

THE SINGLE-BREASTED SUIT

A popular style and is equally effective in Tweeds, Serges, or Pin-striped Worsteds. Our interpretation of this style for this season shows bold, square-cut lapels, and this is unquestionably the correct thing for the well-dressed man. It is tailored to customer's personal measurements and the workmanship is perfect in every detail. Our made-to-measure service assures you of clothes of distinction and quality at distinctly reasonable prices. And our "money-back" guarantee protects you all the time.

PRICES FOR COMPLETE SUITS (Easy Self-measurement Form in centre of this Booklet.)

D.B.			S.B.		
Range A	Men's 42/6	Youths' 39/-	Range A	Men's 40/-	Youths' 36/6
" B	" 47/6	" 43/6	" B	" 45/-	" 41/-
" C	" 55/-	" 51/-	" C	" 52/6	" 48/6
" D	" 62/6	" 58/6	" D	" 60/-	" 56/-
" E	" 70/-	" 65/6	" E	" 67/6	" 63/-
" F	" 82/-	" 77/6	" F	" 79/6	" 75/-

Range Gent's Serge Suitings, 52/6 to 75/- Youths' 48/6 to 71/-
Men's sizes up to 42-inch chest, 40-inch waist, over these measurements 5/- extra.
Youths' sizes up to 33-inch chest, 31-inch waist, over these measurements charged at men's rates.

SHOPPING

The socio-economic growth in the early part of the decade meant that more and more men were able to afford made-to-measure suits. This led to a much wider selection of fashion illustration and advertising in men's periodicals.

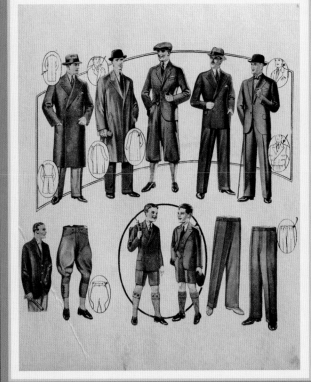

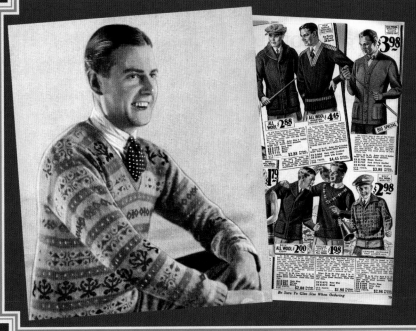

KNITWEAR

With the growing casual attitude towards appearance, knitwear became more avant garde and consequently more visible in men's wardrobes. The Prince of Wales (who later became King Edward VIII and, after his abdication, the Duke of Windsor) had an enormous impact on men's fashion, going as far as to have his portrait painted in a Fair Isle jumper, which drove many fashion-conscious young men to copy his style. Round neck and shawl collars, together with the prototypical V-neck, were all considered correct woollen attire for the modern man.

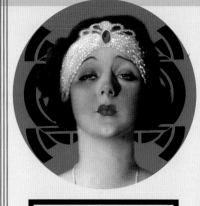

Women's fashions changed almost as fast as musical styles during the 1920s. With the popularity of overseas travel, the wealthy returned with intriguing materials and traditional costumes from abroad. Exotic styles were welcomed by the young, which led to kimonos, harem pants, turbans, cheongsams and many other such outfits gracing the pages of *Harpers Bazaar* and *Vogue*. Leading designers and fashion houses of note that produced designs influenced by these styles include Coco Chanel, Paul Poiret, Elsa Schiaparelli, Callot Souers, Jeanne Lanvin, Jacques Doucet and Madame Tirocchi. As these names suggest, Europe – namely Paris and Italy – was a hub for couture clothing, with the rich and famous flocking to those cities to acquire pieces from limited collections.

Having dominated the previous decade, French fashion designer Paul Poiret was still revered by many. However, his manufacturing standards did not match up to the competition of the time and, by 1929, he was on the brink of bankruptcy. Poiret struggled to come to terms with the popular 'garçonne' look and admitted that his dresses were made only to be 'read beautifully from afar'. This proved to be the downfall of his business, despite championing women's freedom from the constraints of the corset and his draping of fabrics to accentuate the female form, which made his wearable works of art such an important influence during the twenties.

KIMONOS

The traditional Japanese kimono became a central part of Western fashion during the 1920s, with women flocking to wear the silk embroidered gowns. The T-shaped, straight cut of the design was perfect to pair with the style of dresses being worn and the wide-cut sleeves offered an elegant edge for all shapes and sizes. The gowns were of particular appeal to heavier-set ladies with large busts who found it inappropriate to expose the upper arm in spaghetti-strapped flapper dresses.

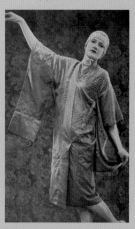

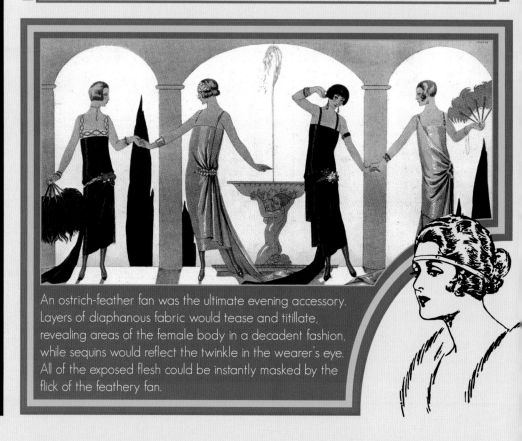

An ostrich-feather fan was the ultimate evening accessory. Layers of diaphanous fabric would tease and titillate, revealing areas of the female body in a decadent fashion, while sequins would reflect the twinkle in the wearer's eye. All of the exposed flesh could be instantly masked by the flick of the feathery fan.

DANCE DIVAS

The dance crazes of the era reflected the optimism of the times. To dance the Charleston, the Black Bottom and the Tango you needed to dress for ease of movement. This was also of vital importance to those taking part in dance marathons, which were all the rage and offered monetary prizes. Busts, bottoms and a belly were often difficult to hide in spaghetti-strapped evening wear. Those with large busts typically resorted to the likes of the Symington Side Lacer, which allowed the wearer to pull strings either side of the bra to flatten the breasts. The less well off took to bandaging their bosoms. Girdles were popular because suspenders were still needed to hold up the stockings, which were now produced in an array of 'nude' colours to emphasize the idea of revealed flesh.

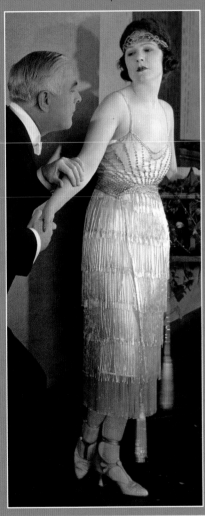

Evening coats, like this Schiaparelli design from 1925, were tailored to reflect the principles of the Art Deco movement. Simple tailoring meant that designs typically had wide collars and a wrap front fastened with a single button or buckle and a hemline that fell just below the knee. The 1920s twist was the dropped waist in line with the top of the hip.

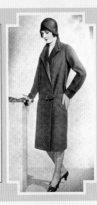

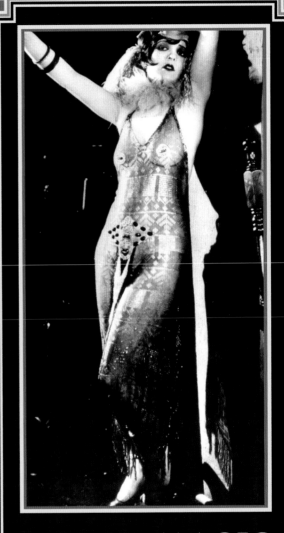

MOVIE MAGIC

By the end of the decade, with the growing film industry in Hollywood, movie actors and actresses became idolized, and fans copied what they wore and how they looked extensively.

The arrival of the first 'talking picture' in 1927 meant that 'silent' starlets like Mary Pickford and Clara Bow (above) made way for 'talking' beauties such as Marlene Dietrich and Greta Garbo, who were creating waves with their style. Pictured in popular movie magazines such as *Photoplay*, *Silver Screen* and *Motion Picture*, these publications became alternative guides to the must-have designs worn by the stars of the day. With the female form only recently unveiled from high necks and low hemlines, some of the flesh-flashing creations being worn created outrage amongst the older generations.

The practical necessity of dressing more simply during the Great War had influenced large-scale changes in men's fashion, with some flexibility being introduced into the guidelines for men's evening wear. Top hat and tails – forever in the lexicon of vintage fashion – remained essential wear for formal occasions in the 1920s. Indeed, the older generation of more aristocratic standing continued to wear a silk top hat for business in the day, while the younger generation were rebelling against that look.

The 1925 edition of the *Vogue Book of Etiquette*, stated that, 'People of the social world are supposed to dress for each other, not for the populace'. Overdressing in public became a matter of social ridicule; nonetheless, it was important to maintain standards. Edward, Prince of Wales, had a reputation for behaving outside the constraints of accepted decorum, and he popularized the tuxedo at the dining table. Other styles included the black worsted single-breasted jacket with a peak lapel or shawl collar with a silk facing in satin. Trousers had to match the jacket in both material and colour, and have a single braid along the seams. Waistcoats were typically white in a U- or V-shape, and shirts were required to have a stiff white plain front with detachable wing or upright collars with single cuffs..

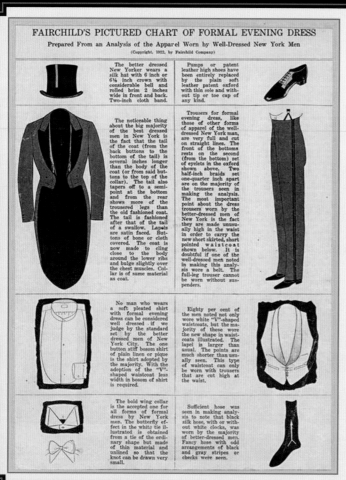

FAIRCHILD'S PICTURED CHART OF FORMAL EVENING DRESS
Prepared From an Analysis of the Apparel Worn by Well-Dressed New York Men
(Copyright, 1922, by Fairchild Company)

GENTS ONLY!

Whether one wore a tailcoat or a dinner jacket, it was essential to add a waistcoat to one's attire. Another 1920s shift was the acceptance of the white waistcoat with the dinner jacket. In fact, this item became a symbol of sartorial elegance after it was sported by two of the most celebrated young men of the day, the Prince of Wales and his cousin, Lord Louis Mountbatten - not to mention a hoard of international aristocrats, socialites and hangers-on who travelled around the glittering cities of the world.

If wealth or social standing was new to you (and you did not have a valet who could provide a dressing service) there were endless charts and handbooks (left) that could help you work out what to wear and how to wear it. Once you had your socks, suspenders, shirt with detachable wing collar, white tie, white waistcoat, trews, tailcoat, patent leather shoes and silk top hat (and perhaps a cane), only then were you considered appropriately dressed as a fashionable man about town! But even then it was imperative that you kept up with ever-changing etiquette regarding men's attire.

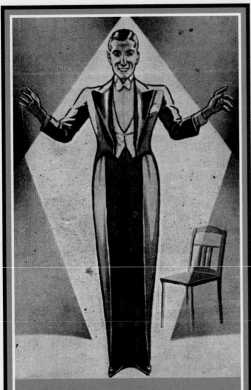

TAILS IT IS!

For formal evening wear tailcoats fell quite short at the front (but no higher than the waistcoat) to reveal a high-waist trouser. Fashion for lapels came and went but the introduction of a little lapel pocket saw the resurgence of the decorative handkerchief.

Get the Look with Hannah

Much like all original garments from this decade, finding men's evening wear undamaged can be hard, although there are plenty of reproductions that are becoming vintage in their own right. It is still fairly easy to find original shirts, often in the original packaging after laundering. However, metal pins would have been used to keep folds in place, so look for rust marks where the pins have been. Also, shirt sizes will generally be similar to a modern classic cut rather than slim fit, which means that the body and tails of the shirt will be wide and long.

TOP TOFF

For the first few years of the decade men dressing for engagements after 6 p.m. often chose to wear rolled collars finished in silk, single-breasted tuxedos or tailcoats fixed at the high-cut front waist by two little cufflink-like chains. Swallow-tail jackets had particularly long tails at the rear. Tippling canes with hollowed-out tops where alcohol could be stored were a novelty and were often specially commissioned with interesting top handle designs made in sterling silver. It was unusual for a man of any class not to smoke, so carrying a cigarette case, usually made of silver or enamel, was integral to the man-about-town look.

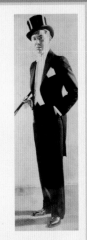

One bastion of the social elite that still demanded the highest standards of dress was the opera. Men were expected to wear a silk top hat, scarf and white gloves. Women that accompanied them often had an opera coat specifically for the occasion. A mix of snobbery and tradition meant that these high-fashion styles were seen in international opera houses throughout most of the twentieth century, but remained out of the reach of all but the fashionable elite.

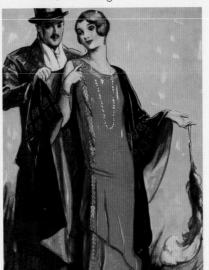

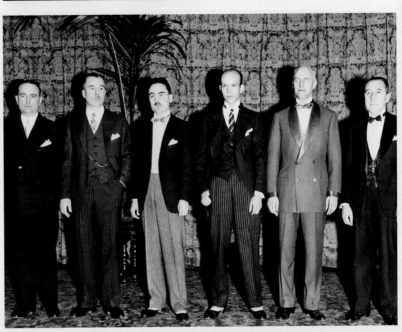

1920s SHOES

With ankles now widely exposed, shoe manufacturers in the twenties went into overdrive to create footwear attractive enough to match the embellished dresses, sturdy enough to dance in and practical enough to walk in. Richard Felton Outcault, the creator of the 'Buster Brown' comic strip, presented a character named Mary Jane at the turn of the century. The American Brown Shoe Company bought a licence from Outcault to use the character of Mary Jane to advertise its products, and a design for a ladies' shoe was given the name Mary Jane. This shoe had a block heel, a rounded closed toe with a simple bar across the bridge of the foot and was fastened with a button. The name has remained to this day. As evening wear demanded ever more glamorous design, ladies favoured the Louis (curved) heel. Those who could afford the luxury had their footwear decorated with tooled patterns or Bargello needlework and sparkling embellishment, which made the shoes works of art in their own right. Fashion footwear for men included the popular Oxford brogues, spats (for the more flamboyant) and one-holed lace-ups in patent leather for the evening. All these styles are now regarded as classics and have been continually copied by designers throughout the decades to the present day.

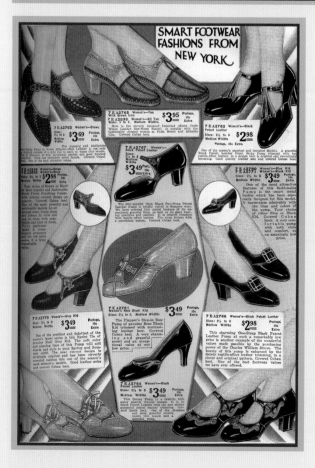

STEPPING OUT

Some women's shoes were made of exotic materials, such as crocodile or snakeskin, or even silk. The truly fashionable had different styles of shoes for different activities: country pursuits, tennis, golf, riding, driving and dancing. Of course, there was always a shoe catalogue to consult for any additional needs.

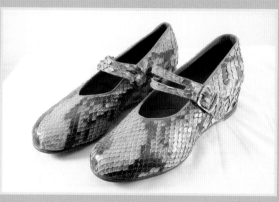

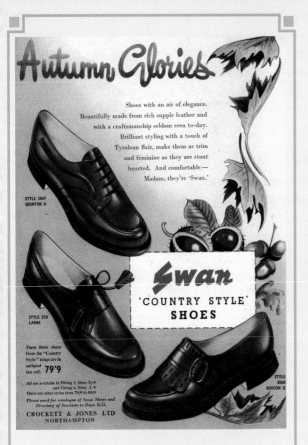

Women's day shoes (above) became more masculine in style as women became emancipated from the house and developed a new awareness of healthy living, involving the pursuit of exercise and fresh air.

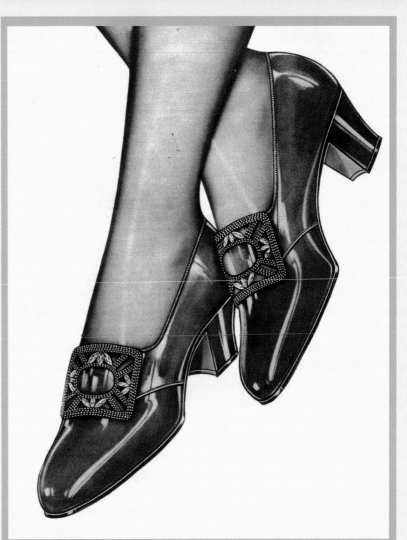

The United Kingdom was famed for its footwear industry, leading the way in technology and development. Shoe manufacturing, based in the towns of Leicester, Kettering and Northampton, employed over a quarter of a million people at one stage.

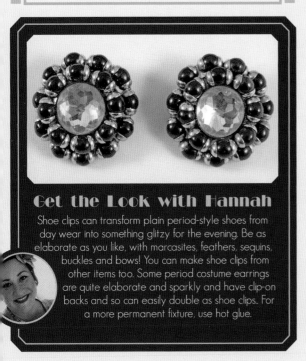

Get the Look with Hannah

Shoe clips can transform plain period-style shoes from day wear into something glitzy for the evening. Be as elaborate as you like, with marcasites, feathers, sequins, buckles and bows! You can make shoe clips from other items too. Some period costume earrings are quite elaborate and sparkly and have clip-on backs and so can easily double as shoe clips.. For a more permanent fixture, use hot glue.

SPARKY!

Men's shoes set the tone for the future with twenties' designs becoming classics. The leather soles of work boots would have been protected by the addition of metal segs, or blakeys. These clearly distinguished the footsteps of a gentleman from those of a working man, whose footwear was noisy and could even cause sparks against the cobblestones.

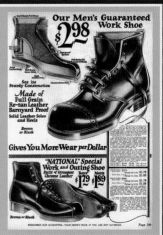

1920s SPORTSWEAR

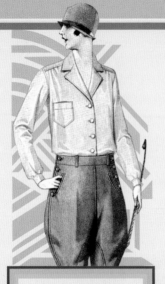

The sudden and popular arrival of sportswear corresponded with the increasing amount of leisure time that many people had to enjoy and the popularization of sport as a healthy pastime. For some the various 'seasons' offered endless possibilities, from skiing in Switzerland in the winter, to rowing at Henley and tennis at Wimbledon in summer, plus the polo season, equestrian events and sailing during Cowes week. Then there was the start of the country sports season from the 'Glorious 12th' of August on British grouse moors. Tennis and golf became more popular with both sexes, and cricket continued to stand the test of time as the archetypal English pursuit. The woman or man about town needed to have the right outfits to follow their hobbies. Sports stars of the day led the way in new sportswear trends: Jean René Lacoste not only became a tennis champion but gave his name to summer sportswear still worn today.

As more women discovered the joys of water sports – including the exciting new option of water-skiing – endless swimsuit designs were created without their Edwardian lengths and layers. The designs revealed as much skin as was permissible in polite society so a suntan was a must have. Coco Chanel had started the craze for sunbathing and the resulting healthy glow when she inadvertently burnt her skin in hot weather.

Tennis took off in a big way in this decade, and special shoes were designed for the players. Made with a canvas lining and leather-covered insoles, they had an extra-thick rubber sole with a ¼-inch (6 mm) heel lift. They were a far cry from the complexities of athletic footwear worn today.

Shoes for Tennis

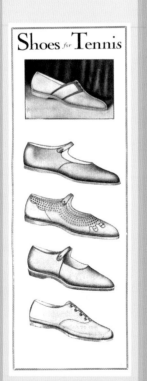

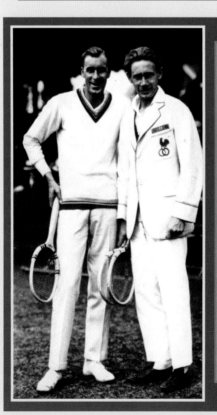

ANYONE FOR TENNIS?

Sportswear from the 1920s set the style for many designers and high-street retailers through to the modern day. These tennis whites (left) would hardly look out of place on the rails of traditional outfitters Hackett or Gant. However, the weight of the fabrics in these original pieces is considerably heavier than those used today. Variations of wool fibre were most commonly used for sportswear as it provided durability. But woollen items often caused problems for the players as they worked up a sweat – their outfits became heavier and more cumbersome the longer they were on the court.

SWIMWEAR

Women had been permitted to compete in swimming events in the 1912 Olympics, and the more relaxed attitude towards the revealing of female flesh allowed swimwear designers in the 1920s to flourish. The American company Jantzen was one of the first manufacturers of the swimsuit, which it promoted with the slogan 'The Suit That Changed Bathing to Swimming'. Until the mid 1930s swimwear was produced in knitted wool, which made the garments incredibly heavy when wet and ensured the bather would never look glamorous once they emerged from the water. The cut of bathing suits was rather standard, generally stopping at mid thigh with attached modesty shorts. Bathing caps for women often resembled cloche hats, which suited the fashion for short hairstyles.

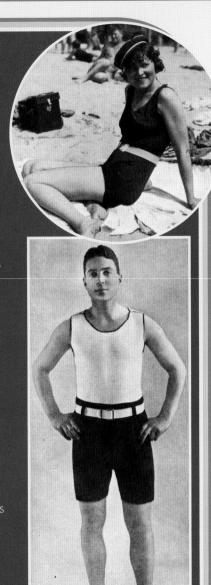

SWING AND BAT

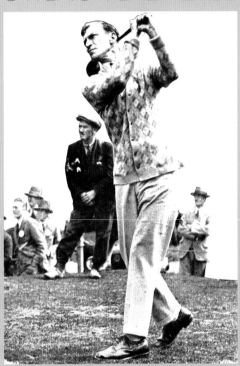

Golf and cricket were very popular outdoor leisure pursuits and sports' outfits were big business. Many fashion-conscious men and women were keen to be seen in the latest designs. Sporting participants were cutting edge in Burberry ladies' free-stroke golf coat, a Best & Co 'Shirtmaker' golf dress or indeed anything in Jean Patou's Sport Et Voyage collection or by Jean René Lacoste. Knitted jumpers and cardigans today considered unisex fashion, were worn by spectators as well as players.

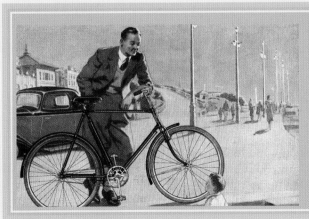

Cycling was very popular, and for gentlemen a pair of plus fours would be the most popular outfit choice. The first Winter Olympics were held in 1924 and they set fashion trends for ladies. Straight pleated skirts were popular on the slopes, although knickerbockers and trousers offered a far more practical option.

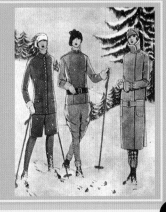

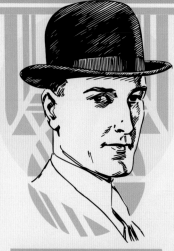

What accessory could be more synonymous with 1920s style than the cloche hat? A couple of years into the decade saw women everywhere cutting their hair into a straight bob or shingle, followed by a mix of both styles called the 'bingle', for the latest pageboy look. Later in the decade an even shorter style, known as the Eton Crop, became popular. And what better way to reveal this new cut than by wearing a hat with a much reduced brim size. Cloches were head hugging and comparatively cheap to make as they needed very little expertise to shape them. Jewellery was much influenced by Art Deco design, and new crazes, such as Egyptomania, kicked off an enthusiasm for 'slave bangles', worn by girls on the upper arm, which accentuated the flesh on display. This exotic look was further heightened by women's tendency to brandish a cigarette holder. However, more demurely, parasols and fans were very popular, as were fur stoles, long silk scarves and the ubiquitous clutch bag.

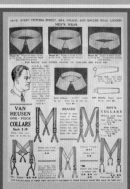

COLLARS & BRACES

Less of an accessory and more of an essential was the detachable collar. All shirts were sold with several collars, which allowed gentlemen to change them according to the occasion. Braces were also worn in a variety of styles and helped to define the look of an outfit.

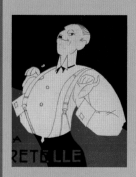

HEADWEAR

The choice of men's headwear was still heavily influenced by class and occupation. It ranged from the top hat, via the more everyday bowler for business or trilby for daywear, down to the lowlier cap. Originally a working man's head covering, the cap was appropriated by the more well to do to finish off their sporting look. Summertime called for a straw boater or a Panama. At the beginning of the 1920s, Homburg hats were worn as an alternative to the bowler but soon the trilby (or fedora), with its creased crown and fabric band took its place in the popularity stakes (especially among Chicago gangsters). The trilby was regarded as a staple of men's fashion for the following fifty years.

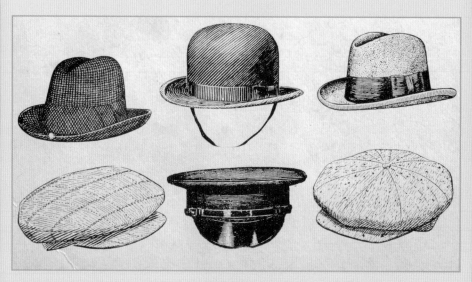

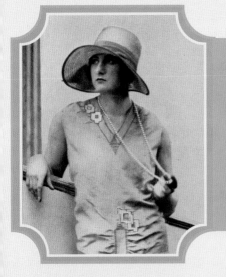

CLASSIC JEWELS

Long beaded necklaces were the accessory worn by many women until, in 1929, *Vogue* pronounced the fashion dead and demanded that pearls and beads were worn shorter once again.

WRAPPED UP

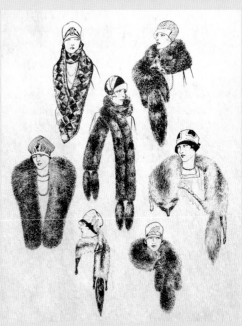

From fur to silk, luxurious materials were placed on or draped around the head, neck or shoulders. These were then usuallly adorned with marcasite or pyrite brooches, scarf ties or hat pins. Europe, America and the UK had their fair share of fine jewellers, such as Cartier, Georg Jensen, Tiffany and Asprey to name but a few.

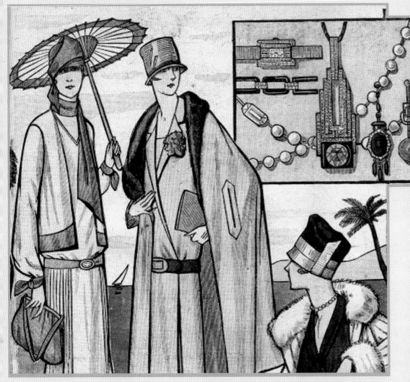

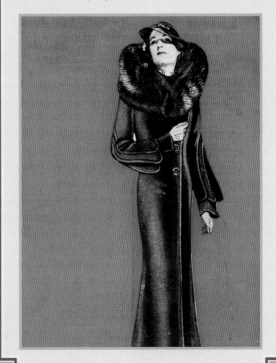

Embellished clutch bags and purses were very important items in a woman's wardrobe. Chainmail purses were all the rage but a more affordable evening design included embroidered fabric, a style that stood the test of time throughout the decade.

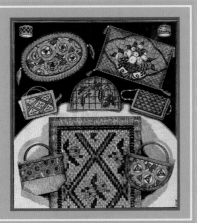

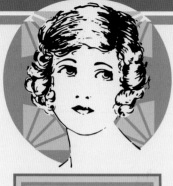

SIZE OF THE 20S

Twenties styling lends itself best to those with lithe limbs and a small bust. This applies equally to menswear as the majority of high-end vintage clothing from this period is sized for gentlemen with a slim frame. It's also worth taking into consideration what you plan to do while wearing original vintage clothing. You might want to wear a larger size than normal for dancing or sports to allow greater freedom of movement.

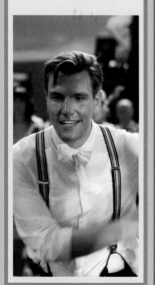

The loss of male lives in World War I meant there was a high ratio of women to men. There was a very real pressure on unmarried women to secure a husband or face the prospect of ending up a childless spinster. This led to a heightened sense of awareness in all

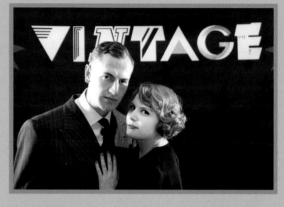

areas of presentation and meant wearing and applying make-up in public became fashionable. Period compacts are highly decorative and were an integral part of any overall look.

Fashion colour palettes generally reflected the pigments that were being discovered through foreign travel, so apart from the all pervasive black, women should look for azure blue, poppy red, bottle green and tangerine orange outfits and accessories. Men tended to choose a more traditional look, so black, ash grey, chestnut brown, Oxford blue and brilliant white should feature heavily.

MEN'S LOOK

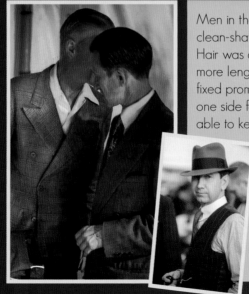

Men in the twenties were either completely clean-shaven or sported a pencil moustache. Hair was a short back and sides with slightly more length on top, styled to the side with a fixed prominent parting or swept back gently to one side for a softer finish. American men were able to keep the hairstyle of choice in place with Murray's Pomade, while the British gent reached for Brylcreem, which was originally developed and manufactured in Birmingham. Both hair product brands have stood the test of time and are still in production today. It was not considered masculine for a man to wear aftershave.

HEAVEN SCENT

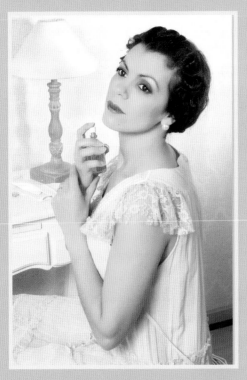

Fragrance was big business for women and nothing says 1920s chic more than Coco Chanel's *No.5*, which was launched in 1921. Enhance the aroma on your skin by using the matching shower gel and body lotion.

Upcycle an evening bag to give it a twenties look. Choose a pouch-shaped plain colour bag with a clasp top and short handle. Then add coloured embroidery, sequins or beads. You can further add tassels, bows or exaggerated fringing to create a totally unique piece.

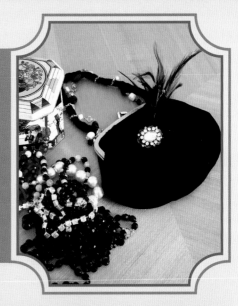

The bandeau is intrinsically linked to the flapper-girl look and works as the perfect accessory to keep hair in place. Typically thicker in width than the more modern-day elasticised headband, the bandeau can be worn plain or bejewelled for either day or evening wear. If you find the bandeau uncomfortable, try wearing the Alice-band style with a sparkly embellished flat motif on one side. If you are feeling creative, make your own for a look that's all yours.

HAIR & BEAUTY

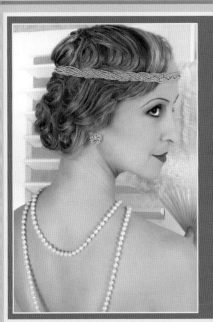

Don't despair if you love the twenties look but you have long hair. It's quite a simple cheat to create with the face-framing styles of the decade by pin curling your locks up, close to your head. Adding a headband can also help to keep your style in place. Remember that the decade focused heavily on the application of cosmetics and that a glow was favourable to a full golden tan. Smokey eye make-up in deep greens and greys with lots of black kohl liner and lashings of mascara accentuated the eyes, and lips were either painted full or minimized 'Geisha' style in deep shades of cranberry and plum to enhance the cupid's bow. Men should stick to a short back and sides hairstyle, but where possible keep the length on top, which should be swept gently back and to the side and kept in place with a good styling wax or pomade, such as 1920s original Black & White.

ASK THE EXPERT

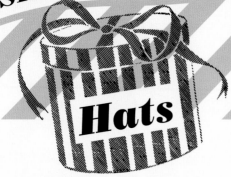

Hats

Quonah Foster is the founder of Maiden Found Millinery. From her studio in North London, she advises on how to buy and care for vintage hats, whether you're buying one for a special outfit or starting a collection.

What types of hats do you collect?

I collect all types of mainstream and unusual hats, headpieces and vintage bridal veils, which I often repair or customize. I have around a hundred pieces. I really love the androgynous and sophisticated look of a trilby or a fedora, but my all-time favourite is the pill box, immortalized by Halston's iconic creation for Jackie Onassis, and the classic percher.

What materials are vintage hats made from?

It depends on the era although felt, straw, silk and wool are most common. As technology progressed and man-made materials grew, a lot of hats and headpieces were made from polyester, nylon and PVC, but the list is endless.

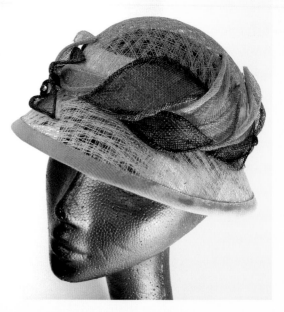

An autumnal windowpane sinamay cloche, with hand-rolled sinamay leaves, reflecting the colours and shapes of the season. Hand blocked using a vintage 1920s hat block.

What are the things to look for when buying a vintage hat?

The first thing I check is the lining. You need to ensure that the lining isn't too damaged as that can affect the overall structure of the piece. Second, check for stains and damage to the exterior of the hat; some damage can be easily rectified. If you see moth holes, walk away!

What is the best way to clean a vintage hat?

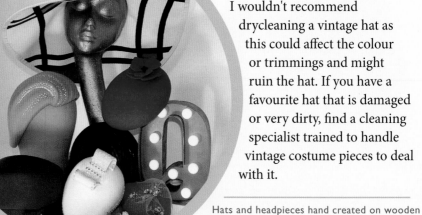

Felt hats are the easiest to clean. Hold the hat over a steaming kettle and brush it gently with a baby's hairbrush. I wouldn't recommend drycleaning a vintage hat as this could affect the colour or trimmings and might ruin the hat. If you have a favourite hat that is damaged or very dirty, find a cleaning specialist trained to handle vintage costume pieces to deal with it.

Hats and headpieces hand created on wooden blocks using traditional techniques inspired by the colours and shapes of different eras.

Can damaged feathers and frills be restored?

If the feathers are soiled I find that a very mild hand soap with lots of water will remove the dirt. Dry the hat naturally and then steam gently to restore the natural shape. With frills, it depends on the damage to the tulle, lace or other material and, of course, your sewing skills as to whether or not these trimmings can be saved. Don't always dismiss a vintage millinery piece because of the condition it is in – even if the trimmings are badly damaged or stained think about ways to rework it, or seek the advice of a good milliner.

What period in history do you think has the most interesting hats and headpieces and why?

That's tricky! The early 1950s had lots of very glamorous headwear and I particularly like the vibrant clashes of colour from the 1960s, which are very exciting. To be honest, I love lots of vintage pieces from different eras but if I had to pick it would probably be the 1940s. During World War II wool was seldom used but lots of other hat materials weren't rationed and embellishments were incredibly creative.

If someone is thinking about collecting hats, what should they start out looking for?

Make sure you start your collection with something you really like – whether it's a particular era, a certain shape, a fabric type or a favourite designer. Just focus on what you are drawn to and feel passionate about rather than something you think has sales value. After that, do your research and scout around. There really is nothing better than finding a gem in a charity shop, vintage fair or even at an auction.

A bespoke bridal headpiece, handmade using traditional methods and decorated with vintage pearls, crystals, silk tulle and ivory felt, encapsulates the personality and individuality of the bride.

What kind of price range can vintage hats fall into?

Many of the materials used in millinery are very attractive to moths and so hats are one of the most common things to find damaged or crumpled, unless they have been stored correctly. This means places like charity shops, thrift shops or car-boot sales will probably only ask a few pounds to keep stock moving and are great places to pick up bargains. Vintage shops may well have taken the time to steam, reshape or repair hats and may well have acquired them in their original hat boxes, which means you could be looking at an average of £20 to £50 per hat. Vintage designer hats such as Dior or Halston can sell for a few hundred pounds but it really depends on where you are buying from. Hats from the 1920s to 1950s in good condition will generally be more sought after than those from the 1960s onwards. However, it is well worth looking out for contemporary designers who have a big following and who will undoubtedly become future vintage.

How should you store vintage hats?

The best place is a hat box with acid-free paper. If you can't find a hat box, any clean box will do but ideally it should be large enough to leave a big gap all around to ensure that the hat is not squashed at any point. Always store your boxes in a dry area away from direct sunlight or excessive moisture.

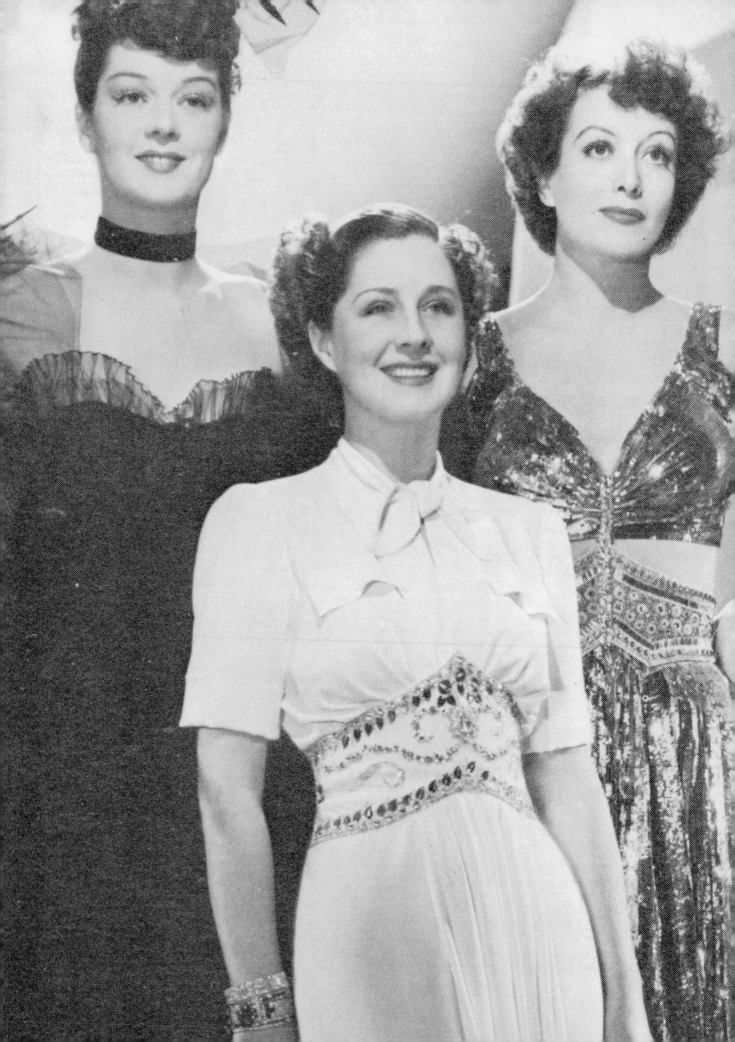

1930s

During the preceding decade, newfound energy and enthusiasm were accompanied by an air of optimism and excitement, which many consumers fuelled by buying on credit. However, lifestyle choices became distinctly more muted for many in the 1930s as the majority of people had to tighten their purse strings owing to the roller-coaster descent of the economy after the Wall Street Crash in 1929 and the dire consequences of the Great Depression that followed. Many people fell into debt and could no longer afford to buy consumer items such as cars and clothes. However how you presented yourself was still of the utmost importance, irrespective of the true state of your finances and this, coupled with the fierce constraints of the class system, continued to define your eligibility for inclusion in certain circles.

In 1936, King Edward VIII abdicated in order to marry American divorcee, Wallis Simpson, and the eyes of the world focused on the pair. Edward, as Prince of Wales, had been something of a trend setter in the 1920s but, with his controversial marriage, fashion and royalty came under closer scrutiny than ever before. Wallis Simpson's sharp dress sense was reported at every opportunity, and Edward and Wallis came to be regarded as one of the most stylish couples of the period. Edward, known as the Duke of Windsor from 1936, favoured American styles that also shaped the fashion choices of many British consumers. The Duke had a fondness for bold patterns and colour, adopting a more relaxed approach to formal occasions, which meant a preference for midnight blue over black for evening wear, as well as a penchant for wearing an extra-large knot in his tie that came to be known as the 'Windsor knot'. Hollywood films and the stars (such as Rosalind Russell, Norma Shearer and Joan Crawford, left) continued to influence both style and standards, from the young and beautiful through to the elegance and sophistication of the more mature.

In 1930, Darryl F. Zanuck, the newly appointed production head of Warner Brothers film studio, made it no secret that his production policy would reflect headline news, bringing the 'gangster' film to centre stage and with it a controversial style of dress and morals. In *Panama Flo* (1932), for example, Helen Twelvetrees' character positively flaunted that it was acceptable to have ill-gotten gowns and furs, so long as you didn't enjoy them. Cutting edge fashion didn't elude the working classes; however haute couture was only accessible to those who could actually afford it and who had the occasion to wear it.

1930s WOMEN'S
Day Wear

During the 1930's economic slump, spending on clothes was drastically reduced. Home dressmaking became more popular, making fashion more accessible. Waistlines for day wear returned to their correct anatomical position, hemlines dropped to the calf, and garments favoured the short trumpet, leg-of-mutton and bishop sleeve. Sophistication was the overriding leitmotif for most designers and this included the trouser suit, cut to accentuate the shoulder width and flatter the hip curves with a wide leg.

SUPERBLY STYLED FROCKS!

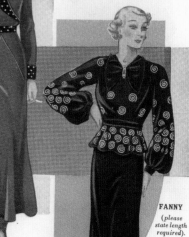

FLORA.
Here is a very striking and charmingly designed Afternoon Frock, with a style appeal that is irresistible. A lovely quality **ART SILK MAROCAIN** is used and a box pleated Coatee effect is incorporated over a pretty figured bodice. The easy fitting sleeves have the popular gauntlet cuffs and the flared skirt has a graceful frill in front.
In ROSE RED as illustration.
In WOMEN'S Size only.
Lengths 48 or 50 ins.

Please state length required. **PRICE 17'11**

FLORA.

FANNY
(please state length required).

PRICE

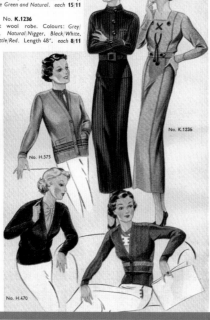

KNITWEAR

Knitwear became a focus, with actress Lana Turner's 1937 film *They Won't Forget*, making her the first 'sweater girl'. Knitwear became part of an acceptable, informal look for young women, which continued to be influential into the 1950s. Knitwear as 'fashion' in the 1930s was arguably the first major youth style movement. Retail stores had dedicated knitwear departments with typical colour palettes favouring teal, brown and bottle green. Home knitting and knitwear patterns also grew in popularity.

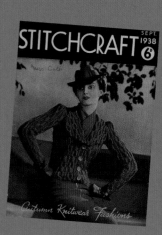

STITCHCRAFT SEPT. 1938 6

Autumn Knitwear Fashions

KNITWEAR DEPARTMENT

"PHILIS" KNITWEAR

No. G.220
Ribbed Suit, lumber coat style with contrasting wool lacings and breast pockets. Colours: Navy, Nigger, Fawn, Bottle Green and Natural. each 15/11

No. K.1236
Women's fine-knit wool robe. Colours: Grey/Red, Nigger/Gold, Natural/Nigger, Black/White, Navy/White and Bottle/Red. Length 48". each 8/11

No. H.575
Scotch-knit Cardigan, with two pockets. Colours: Navy, Wine, Silver Grey, Dark Brown, Light Brown, Dark Blue, Rust and Black. Wms. each 5/11

No. H.574
O.S. Size: each 6/11

No. H.470
Fancy lace-knit Cardigan, welted at waist and cuffs. Colours: Light Beige, Nigger, Red, Navy, Flannel Grey and Black. dozen 47/11

No. H.442
Fancy knitted Cardigan welted waist and cuffs. Colours: Saxe, Wine, Grey, Fawn, Navy, Nigger and Black. doz. 35/11

No. G.220

No. K.1236

No. H.575

No. H.470

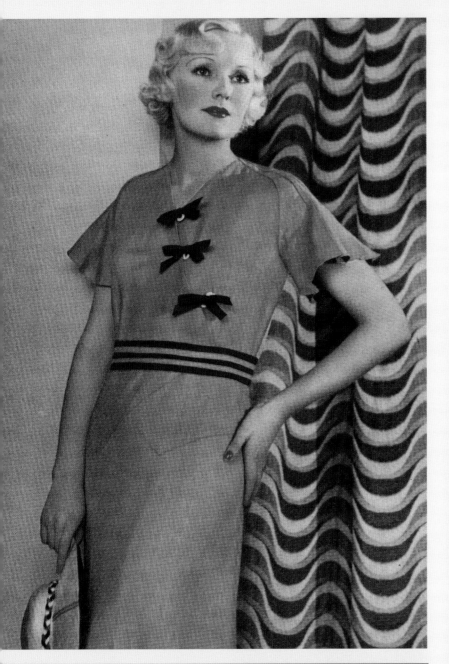

FABRICS

The use of man-made fibres in fabric construction became increasingly popular during the thirties. Previously, silk, cotton and wool were favoured in haute couture tailoring. However, with designers electing to push the fashion boundaries in their quest for exclusivity, rayon and newly developed nylon (1938) were introduced as a point of difference. Both fabrics could be knitted or woven, and rayon provided a cheaper alternative to silk.

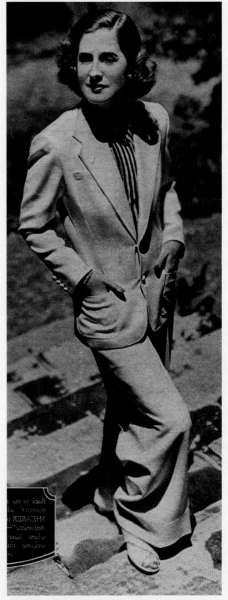

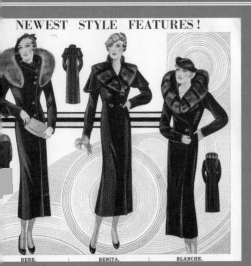

NEWEST STYLE FEATURES !

TRIMS

Fur was the ultimate trim on coats and accessories. Collars, cuffs, hats, muffs and gloves were all made from or finished in fur, with a stole providing the ultimate shoulder drape. Sable, mink, musquash, fox and racoon were some of the pelts in vogue, but more exotic species were also used.

BEBE.   BENITA.   BLANCHE.

1930s MEN'S *Day Wear*

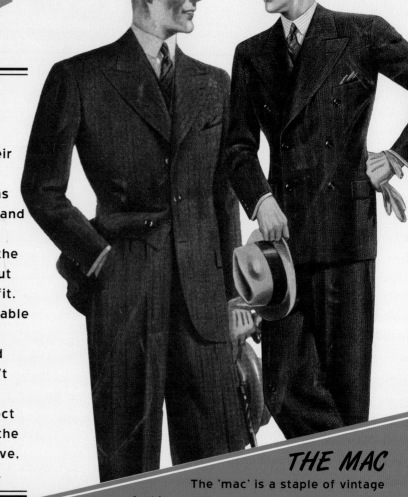

Men's fashions continued to maintain an air of formality regardless of social standing, and young men mostly dressed like their fathers. Working-class men might have had less variety but a suit was compulsory, even if only for work and Sunday best. Drape, reefer, lounge and plus fours were just a few of the styles a man could choose from, but the most important issue was the fit. Shirts were often sold with detachable collars, while ties, much shorter in length than we see now, were held in place with a tie pin so they didn't escape the ubiquitous waistcoat. Fedoras were considered the perfect accessory for day wear, although the trilby and boater were an alternative, as was the working man's flat cap.

THE MAC

The 'mac' is a staple of vintage fashion and none more so than the 1930s version. The Mackintosh was originally developed in 1824 as a waterproof overcoat and briefly had a rival in the form of the 'trench' coat which, as the name suggests, was designed to protect soldiers from the elements in the trenches during World War I.

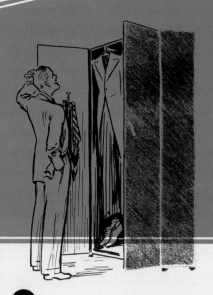

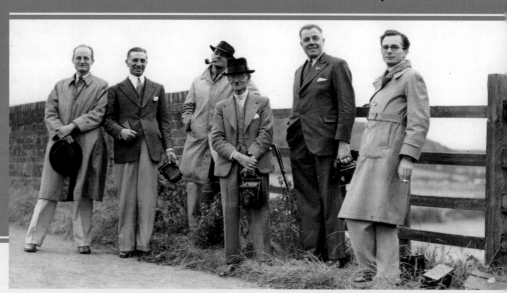

REEFER SUITS

JACKET Two or three buttons. Browns, greys, blues and mixtures. Double breasted lapels, soft rolling, broad chested, snuggly fit on waist and narrow hips.

WAISTCOAT Two or three buttons. Browns, greys, blues and mixtures. Double breasted lapels, soft rolling, broad chested, snuggly fit on waist and narrow hips.

TROUSERS Turn-up, to match jacket.

SHIRT Exactly as worn with single-breasted lounge suit.

COLLAR Double collar, soft, to match shirt, or white collar with self-coloured or white shirt.

TIE Club, school or regimental ; stripes, silks, foulards and poplin in fancy designs.

GLOVES Washable chamois, fawn or yellow.

FOOTWEAR Brown or black shoes according to suit.

HEADWEAR Soft felt hat, either "full framed" or with the modern narrow snap-brim. A black bowler hat is correct with a dark suit.

LOUNGE SUITS

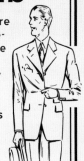

JACKET Three-button, centre button to button, with single- or double-breasted lapel. The shoulders are now "natural" and, in fine tailoring, slightly sloping. The coat is smartly waisted ; should have narrow sleeves, four buttons on the cuff are the fashion now ; and in the latest models an outside ticket pocket is shown.

WAISTCOAT To match, single-breasted, with the last button unfastened.

TROUSERS With turn-ups ; although trousers worn without turn-ups are equally correct.

SHIRT The soft-fronted shirt, coloured or striped, with colour to match, is the fashion. The double collar is greatly favoured as are the double cuffs.

TIE Here individuality enters. The tie should be in tone with the colour of the suit and shirt, or else be in striking contrast.

HEADWEAR The soft hat is really the most appropriate with a light coloured suit. For a dark coloured suit, the black bowler is recommended.

PLUS FOUR SUIT

JACKET Here are a great many different designs from which to select, made up in Scotch or fancy tweeds, checks and herringbone patterns. The single-breasted two or three-button jacket with ordinary pockets, shaped on easy lines, in undoubtedly very good form.

WAISTCOAT Usually a pullover is worn in place of a waistcoat.

PLUS FOURS Should be fairly long and full.

SHIRT Twill, poplin or flannel.

COLLAR To match.

TIE Foulards, wool or wool mixtures of fancy designs.

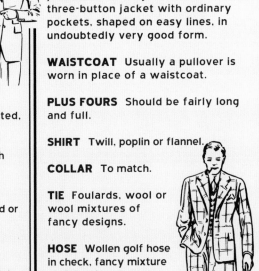

HOSE Wollen golf hose in check, fancy mixture or ribbed in colours to match the suit.

GLOVES Wollen or string gloves when needed.

HEADWEAR Snap-brim, soft felt or cap.

Tall & stout. Corpulent. Average. Tall & slim.   Sloping shoulders.   Medium shoulders.   Square shoulders.

E   F   G

TYPES OF FIGURES

To guide us in cutting your pattern please fill in with a ·X the lines which apply to your figure.

A.................. B.................. C.................. D..................
E.................. F.................. G..................

A   B   C   D

1   2   3   4   5

CUTTING EDGE

The tailoring of men's jackets in the 1930s created a slightly higher waistline than seen previously and trouser legs were distinctly narrower. However, this sometimes varied depending on the overall cut of the suit. Hollywood stars Fred Astaire and Cary Grant in particular were noted for their dapper style and those with more expensive and flamboyant tastes looked to the likes of gangster Al Capone for style inspiration.

Get the Look with Hannah

A cane was an essential accessory. Canes were not merely walking aids but were also a measure of a gentlemen's success and stature. Men would have canes for day, evening and special occasion, fashioned from a variety of materials, and can be extremely collectable in the modern market.

1930s WOMEN'S
Evening Wear

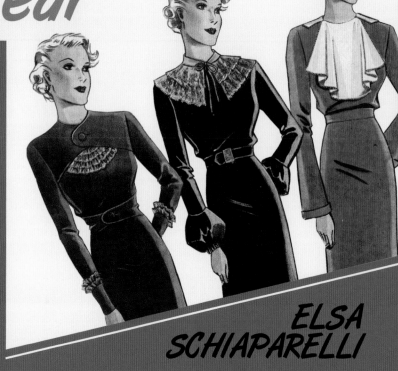

The widespread austerity of the 1930s did not curtail the desire for glamour when it came to women's evening wear. Certain areas of a woman's body, such as the arms, shoulders, décolletage and back, were all highlighted by fashion design during this period. The likes of screen siren Mae West (below) sought to push the boundaries to the extremes with her highly sexualized and provocative dress sense, which became her trademark.

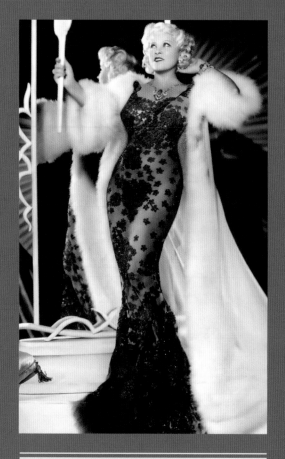

ELSA SCHIAPARELLI

Elsa Schiaparelli was revered in women's fashion throughout the 1930s, experimenting with man-made materials and using her love of surrealist art to influence her designs. Famous for her innovative 'bias cut', her dresses ran sinuously along feminine curves further emphasized by the use of materials such as duchesse satin, crepe de chine and chiffon, which were beautifully hand embellished with beads and sequins. Always looking for ways to push the fashion boundaries, Schiaparelli's signature colour of shocking pink was both a bold and brilliant choice, helping her designs to stand out from the typically subdued tones of the time.

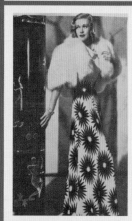

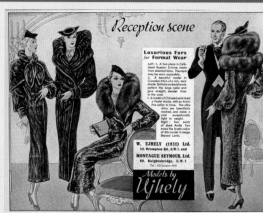

ART & DESIGN

The 1930s was the first time art had a great influence on fashion, with movements such as Art Deco, Cubism and Surrealism inspiring design and the embellishments that adorned the clothes. Artists such as Salvador Dalí, Pablo Picasso, Wassily Kandinsky and Paul Delvaux all used pattern, texture and colour to create abstract paintings, theatre and film sets, and these were replicated in fabric prints and colour palettes throughout the period.

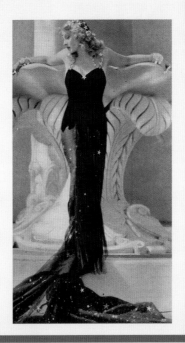

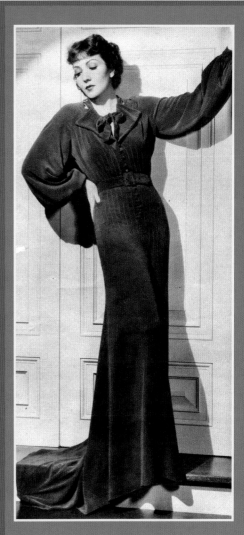

ON THE TOWN

In the 1930s, 'talking pictures' provided a new form of entertainment. For a trip to the 'movie house' formal dress standards were slightly relaxed. However, to attend the theatre, traditional etiquette was maintained, with ladies draped in their most exquisite finery. Jeanne Lanvin was very much in tune with the atmosphere of the time, and her designs maintained an extremely elegant line. Trains on evening dresses became a popular feature and required the wearer to don high-heeled shoes.

VELVET VIXENS

The weight and cut of an evening gown determined how figure hugging it would be and how much movement would be achieved by the wearer. Pile-weave velvet was a sumptuous and expensive fabric choice in the 1930s. It had been used as a luxury material for many decades but, like rayon, proved to be a favourite of high-end designers during the decade. Since it was a difficult fabric to handle, repairs and alterations were awkward to carry out, so precise measurements of the circumference of a high neckline as well as the cuffs, sleeves and waistlines were imperative. This ensured the owner was all too aware of the implications of an expanding physique!

STYLISH TOUCHES

The little black dress was a staple of a woman's wardrobe. Synonymous with Chanel's evening chic, it was the polar opposite of the newly emerging print dress. However, the biggest style change was the arrival of the backless evening dress. Fairly high at the front with a low back cut almost to the waist, it was worn with strings of beads down the spine. Fur continued to be made into bolero coats, capes and shrugs to complete the look archetypal debutante's look.

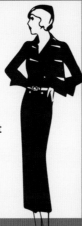

1930s MEN'S
Evening Wear

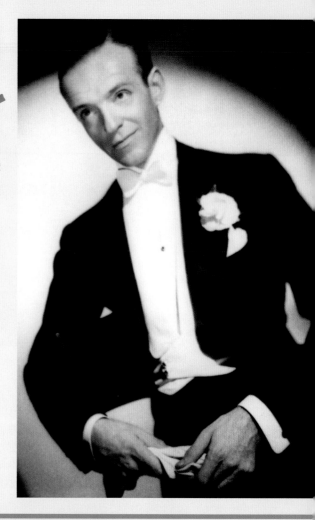

Staying abreast of the latest full dress fashion was of particular importance to gentleman in the 1930s, if for no other reason than because the eminently stylish Prince of Wales was being photographed at every opportunity for a plethora of men's periodicals. The prince was ranked alongside actors Fred Astaire (right), James Cagney and Errol Flynn for his debonair dress sense and dashing good looks, becoming something of a feature on the celebrity social circuits in the UK, Europe and the USA. Also, as transatlantic travel increased opulent ocean liners required a very specific dress code to be maintained for evening wear and getting it wrong could mean social stigmatization.

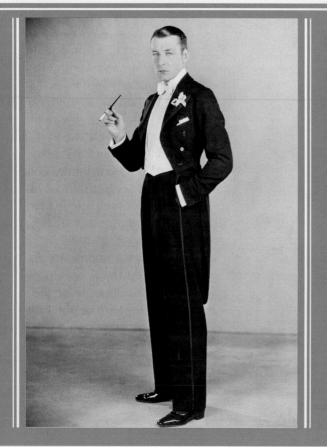

SMART ELEGANCE

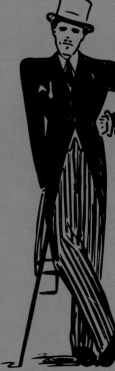

In the early 1930s, there were two distinct styles of evening tailcoats. The American coat had a slightly lower waist, natural shoulders and no excess material. In contrast, the British style featured a high waist and wide shoulders with lots of extra fullness across the chest and around the shoulder blades. The British look gradually dominated as a result of its patronage by the Prince of Wales (before 1936), whose tailor favoured a short lapel to create a vertically elongating effect. False cuffs, no breast pocket and silk cloth buttons instead of bone were other popular trends from London's exclusive West End during the early 1930s.

BLACK COAT AND STRIPED TROUSERS

IS THE IDEAL AND CORRECT WEAR FOR SOLICITORS AT COURT, THE MEDICAL MAN, THE STOCKBROKER AND, IN FACT, FOR ALL PROFESSIONAL AND BUSINESS MEN, WHO HAVE TO APPEAR NEATLY AND SUITABLY DRESSED IN THE RESPECTIVE VOCATIONS AND YET DO NOT FEEL THE NEED OF WEARING A MORNING COAT

OVERCOAT   A dark grey or black chesterfield or a dark grey double-breasted Guards coat.

WAISTCOAT   Black, single breasted.

TROUSERS   Striped with no turn-ups.

SHIRT   The soft-fronted shirt, coloured or striped, with colour to match, is the fashion. The double collar is greatly favoured as are the double cuffs.

COLLAR   White double, soft to match shirt

TIE   Black

GLOVES   Wash Leather

HOSE   Black Cashmere or Silk

FOOTWEAR   Brown or black shoes according to suit

HEADWEAR   Black bowler

MORNING COAT

FOR FORMAL OCCASIONS SUCH AS WEDDINGS, FUNERALS, GARDEN PARTIES, LUCHEONS

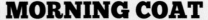

COAT   One-button black coat, single or double-breasted lapels. Smartly waisted, with narrow four-button sleeves and fairly long tails. The grey coat in a light or dark shade is frequently worn to luncheons, garden parties ect.

WAISTCOAT   For all festive occasions, a plain light grey, light lavender or even light fawn vest is permissible; single or double breasted, buttons to match. With grey morning coat the vest should be either light grey or white. Fancy designs in vests are bad taste. For funerals, a black single-breasted vest.

TROUSERS   Striped or checked cashmere, cheviots or worsteds; no turnups. With grey morning coat the trousers should be of the same material. For funerals, only dark striped trousers should be worn.

SHIRT   Soft white, popin or silk with soft or semi-soft fronts. (Coloured shirts or shirts of any kind are very bad form.)

COLLAR   Square wing or double collar

TIE   Open-end tie to match vest with neat black or grey pattern. No vivid colours should be used.

GLOVES   Wash leather.

HOSE   Plain black silk, cashmere or mercerised

FOOTWEAR   Black patent leather, lace up shoes.

HEADWEAR   Black or grey top hat.

EVENING WEAR

FOR DINNER PARTIES AND CLUB USE

DINNER JACKET   Either single-breasted or double-breasted in black or midnight blue. The double-breasted is usually a two-button coat, with only the lower button fastened.

For Dances, theatre, dinner-parties, ect., when ladies are present **THE FULL DRESS SUIT** is the only correct wear.

WAISTCOAT   A Black vest, "V" shaped with three buttons. The ultra-modern young man has adopted the white vest with black buttons. There is really nothing incorrect about it, although it is not a style for the elderly man. The full dress tail coat, however, is always worn with a white pique or vest, either single or double breasted.

TROUSERS   To match coat style; single row of braid with the dinner jacket and a double row with tails.

SHIRT   With the dinner suit, a soft or semi-soft front is permissible; with the double-breasted jacket, it is necessity, or else it is difficult to sit. With full dress, a stiff linen or pique shirt is the correct wear. In both cases the cuffs are stiff.

COLLAR   Wing or turn-down collar for the dinner suit, but for evening dress only the wing collar is correct

TIE   Black for dinner suit; white for evening

GLOVES   Wash leather for outdoor and theatre wear. White kid for dances only.

HOSE   Plain black silk.

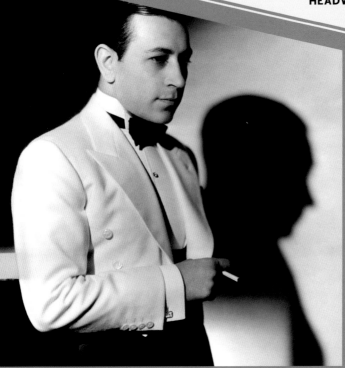

ALL WHITE ON THE NIGHT...

White dinner jackets were originally seen on fashion-conscious gentlemen in warm climates during the thirties. They were mostly constructed in light fabrics (linen, cotton drill or silk) and combined with either black or white trousers and a black bow tie. Traditional buttonhole decoration choices ranged from a white gardenia or carnation, to a red carnation as favoured by the Prince of Wales.

1930s *Shoes*

Men's and women's shoe designs had become more graceful by the 1930s. The continued popularity of dancing meant the ankles and feet of both sexes were still very much in focus. The heels of women's shoes shifted away from the more cumbersome Louis XIV heel and turned into the precursor for the stiletto. As hemlines on dresses extended downwards during the decade, there was a need for height to elongate the body and carry off the *en-vogue* fan-tailed skirts or dress trains. As with men's clothing trends, formal shoes followed a distinct path; elegant and sophisticated or gangster chic. The increase in popularity of different sports also created a need for footwear to accommodate activities from golf and tennis to skiing and ice-skating.

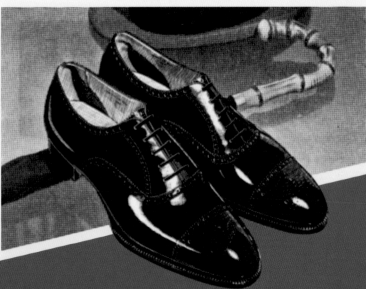

Get the Look with *Hannah*

A dapper thirties male would never allow his shoes to show him up. Invest in a good polishing kit and make sure that your toes and heels do not become scuffed or worn. Purchase a good set of shoe stretchers too; these will help you to avoid creases and mis-shapen leather.

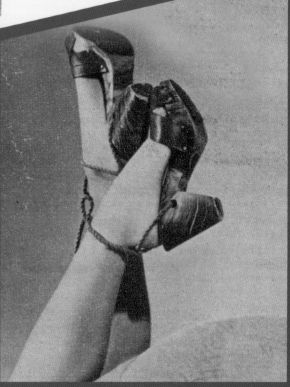

CORKED!

By the mid thirties, political unrest was starting to affect the availability of shoe materials in Italy. This had a serious impact on the work of famed shoe designer Salvatore Ferragamo and prompted him to make innovative use of unconventional materials in his designs. Cork soles, historically used to make Italian and Spanish chopines (16th-century shoes with very high wooden or cork soles) provided height and stability and were functional, allowing Ferragamo to present the modern 'platform' shoe. The style immediately became popular throughout Europe and North America.

BROGUES

This plain style of gentlemen's leather lace-up was the shoe of choice throughout the twenties and thirties when brogues became the height of fashion. The Oxford brogue was also a lace-up but with multiple leather pieces perforated and serrated to create a decorative pattern. There were many perforation styles including the full brogues (UK) or wingtips (USA) with multiple perforations around the entire shoe. Half brogues were designed by famous British shoemaker John Lobb in 1937 as an alternative to the plain Oxford or quarter brogue.

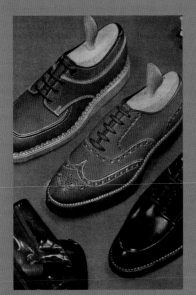

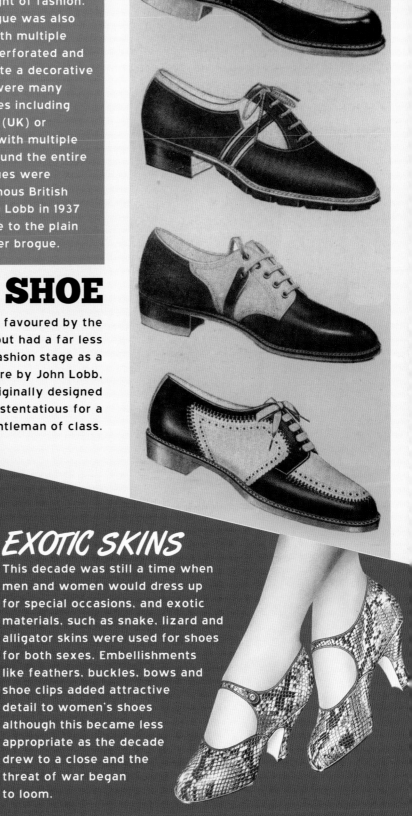

SPECTATOR SHOE

This shoe was most famously favoured by the flamboyant gangster Al Capone but had a far less controversial inauguration to the fashion stage as a sport's shoe design. Brought to the fore by John Lobb, the spectator shoe (right) was originally designed for cricket but thought too ostentatious for a gentleman of class.

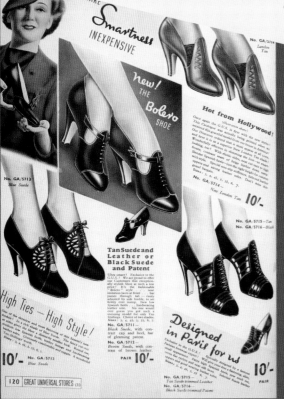

EXOTIC SKINS

This decade was still a time when men and women would dress up for special occasions, and exotic materials, such as snake, lizard and alligator skins were used for shoes for both sexes. Embellishments like feathers, buckles, bows and shoe clips added attractive detail to women's shoes although this became less appropriate as the decade drew to a close and the threat of war began to loom.

1930s *Sportswear*

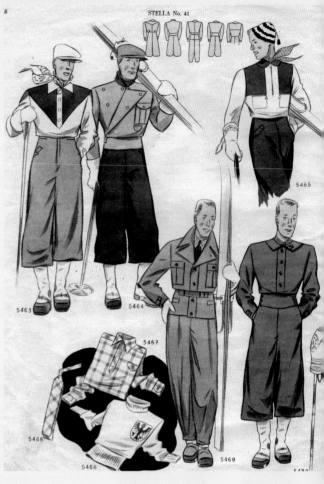

Before the 1930s, sports clothing fell into the functional rather than the fashionable category and was disregarded by acclaimed designers. But during this decade, sporting activities such as tennis, golf, cricket and swimming had become so celebrated that designs for different sporting outfits were gracing the front cover of *Vogue*. With the attraction of the Winter Olympics and skiing becoming *de rigeur* for the upper classes, skiwear also grew increasingly popular. As the demand for sports haute couture increased and a growing number of wealthy individuals had to dress themselves without the assistance of a maid or valet, practical clothing became a necessity. The development of sports fashion coincided with the availability of new synthetic fibres, which were used in sportswear design to facilitate movement and aid performance.

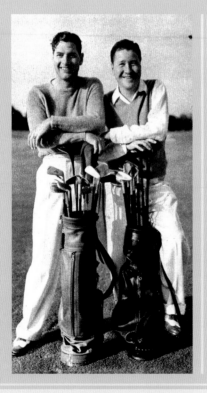

KNIT KIT

Braemar was well established by the 1930s as a manufacturer of hosiery, but it was the company's knitted sportswear that found fame during this decade. Golf was a sport of elegance, and men moved away from knickerbockers and plus fours, choosing instead full-length trousers, which a few would still elect to tuck into long socks. The game was enjoyed by both sexes with separates becoming a category of clothing that grew in importance during the period.

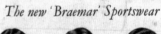

The new 'Braemar' Sportswear

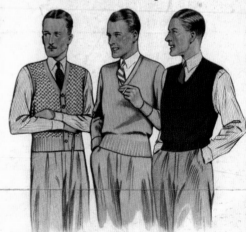

The New 'Waistcotite'
Obtainable in a wide choice of designs after the style of the above. Botany Worsted, in shades of Nigger/Fawn; Blue/Fawn; Brown/Fawn/Yellow; Tan/Fawn/White; Nigger/Blue/Fawn; Grey/Black/White. Sizes 36 to 44 in. Price 17/6

'Taynuilt' Sports Pullover
In Pure Cashmere, light yet warm, soft yet durable. All colours fast. In shades of Grey, Navy, Saxe, Natural, Hunting Yellow, Fawn, Snuff Brown, Mist Blue Mixture. Sizes 36 to 44 in. Price . . . 29/6

'Leyden' Waistite
A close-fitting Pullover in the new light-weight Cashmere, wonderfully soft and warm. In shades of Grey, Light Navy, Natural, Mist Blue Mixture, Nigger, Saxe, Burgundy, Navy. Sizes 36 to 44 in. 21/-

GREENSMITH DOWNES, LTD.
133 George Street, EDINBURGH   1 Bell Street, ST ANDREWS

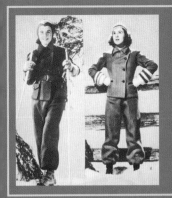

The attraction for alpine skiing was fuelled by the glamour of the resorts. The Winter Olympics of 1932 (Lake Placid, New York) and 1936 (Bavaria, Germany) highlighted prominent female athletes alongside their male counterparts. Suddenly, ski fashions did not require skis and were worn year round for all activities from snow fights to shopping.

TENNIS

Tennis wear became far more practical in the 1930s. As interest in the sport increased, gentlemen ditched heavy flannel trousers in favour of shorts, which gave much more freedom of movement. Women's fashion followed suit, and pleats began to be added to tennis skirts, although the length was still extremely modest compared to today's outfits. Despite these changes, ladies were not allowed to wear shorts for competitions at Wimbledon until 1934, while the men had to wait until 1946.

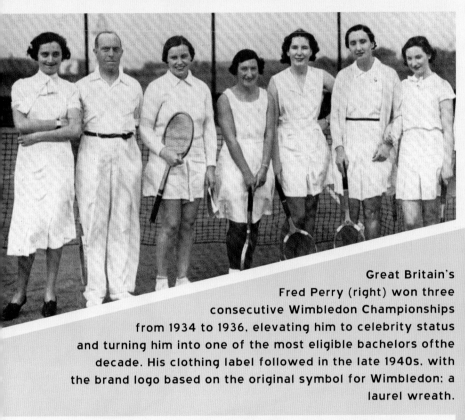

Great Britain's Fred Perry (right) won three consecutive Wimbledon Championships from 1934 to 1936, elevating him to celebrity status and turning him into one of the most eligible bachelors of the decade. His clothing label followed in the late 1940s, with the brand logo based on the original symbol for Wimbledon: a laurel wreath.

ICE QUEEN

Figure skating was still a relatively new phenomenon as a serious sport, having been introduced to the main arena in the first Winter Olympics in 1924. Sonja Henie, a Norwegian champion figure skater and later film star, became the poster girl for both her physical ability and her choice of short skirts to demonstrate her skills. Less athletic and more fashion-conscious young women took to wearing two-piece knitted skirt suits with mittens, and bouclé skating dresses which would flair when twirled.

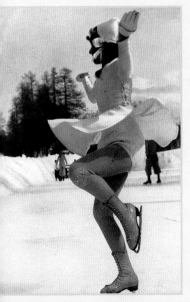

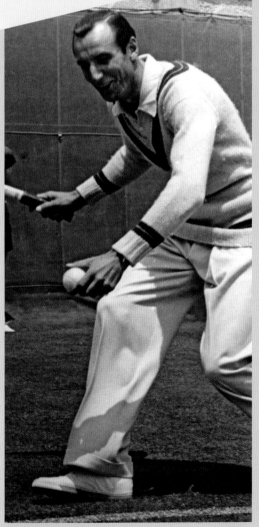

1930s *Accessories*

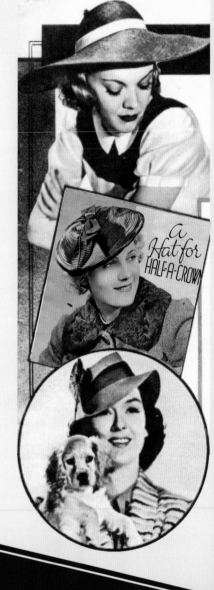

Accessories are usually the affordable way of changing the overall look of an outfit. However, with most people finding the Depression pinching at any spare income, adorning existing outfits with cheaper costume jewellery and other inexpensive items was one way of minimizing outlay. From hats, gloves and sunglasses to handbags and jewellery, the retail market was awash with options. Even first-class travellers on transatlantic liners began switching their priceless gems for faux alternatives. Ladies' hat designs remained delicate and small for most of the decade, with larger brimmed styles becoming popular later on in the thirties. Turbans and berets featured on Hollywood starlets, but the pill-box was the overriding shape of the decade.

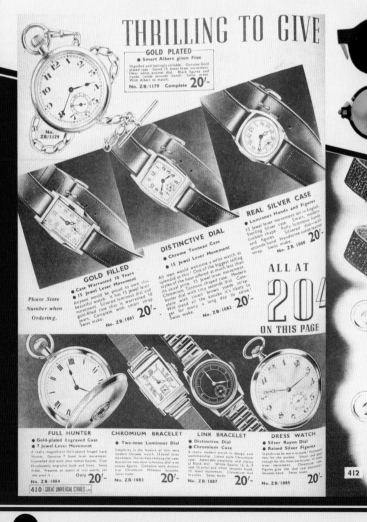

TIME FOR CHANGE

The demand for small, precision watches saw the end of the fob watch in the 1930s. Men's watches were accurate timepieces unlike the female equivalent, which were largely regarded as jewellery. The slimline wrist watch demonstrated advanced technology and a new watch reflected prosperity. There was a trend for rectangular and tonneau-shaped watches, which allowed large components to be transferred from pocket watches into narrow wrist watches.

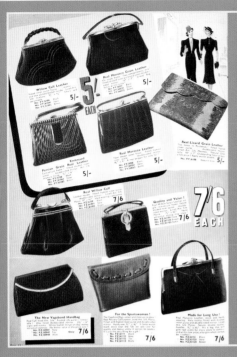

GLOVES AND BAGS

Most women wore gloves when they left the house. These were fabric or leather and worn to the wrist for day wear, and elbow length to complement an evening dress. Gloves were carefully chosen to match shoes and handbags. Day bags became larger during the decade, with both shoulder and clasp bags becoming popular. Many bags reflected Art Deco designs and shapes. For the evening, a small embellished clutch bag was preferred.

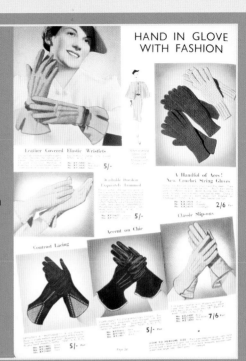

HAND IN GLOVE WITH FASHION

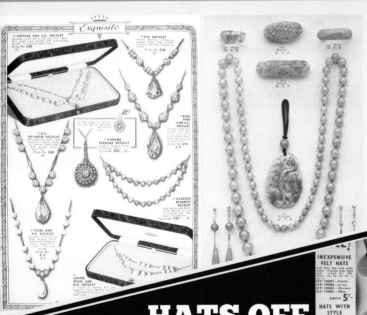

The manufacture of simulated gemstones went into overdrive in the 1930s as the public could no longer afford precious jewels or were forced to sell their existing ones. Silver and pewter-based costume jewellery was made by sought-after designers like Coco Chanel. Jade, widely imported for jewellery in the 1920s, continued to be popular in the thirties, complementing the preferred colour palette of the day.

HATS OFF

There is very little difference between fedora and trilby hats, which were the main options for the dapper gent. Fundamentally, the fedora had a wider brim and a higher crown than the trilby, with the brim of the latter typically being tipped up at the rear. The Homburg was the gentleman's evening hat whilst the flat cap was universally worn by the working-class man. Men also accessorized with gloves, which were usually white synthetic material or chamois leather for evening wear and all leather or leather and cotton palmed for the day.

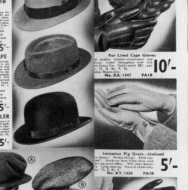

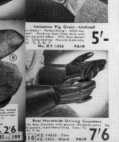

STYLE · COMFORT · QUALITY

1930s *Get the Look with Hannah*

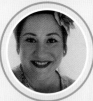

People of most shapes and sizes can find an element of the thirties to embrace, although with fashion veering towards the natural silhouette of both men and women, many designs were made for slim physiques. During the early years, bright colours were celebrated: primrose yellow, mint and bottle green, brick red, sapphire, coral and midnight blue were fashion favourites. Later, more subdued and muted pastels were used alongside pink and duck egg blue with neutral tones taking over. The 1930s was a time of smart presentation so when shopping for thirties styles, look for an accurate fit or consider having garments altered.

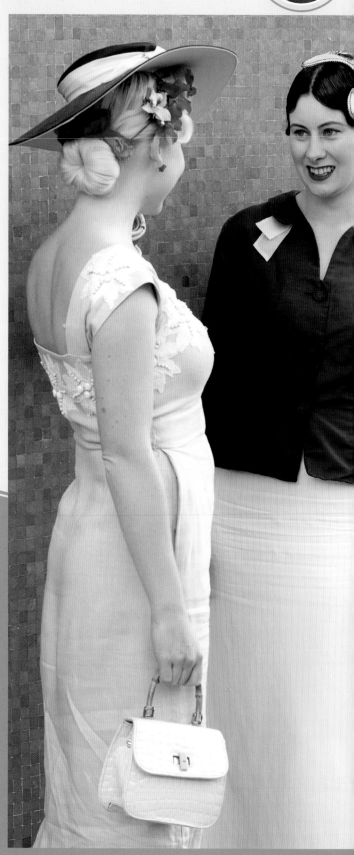

WOMEN'S LOOK

Simplicity and elegance echo through the decade so avoid fussy styles and go for fluid, clean lines. Gloves and delicate small-face wrist watches are a nice touch, and remember that bags were not worn on the shoulder. Your face shape will dictate the most appropriate hat, so bear in mind that a more rounded face will become more balanced with a wide, tall hat, and a slim face will suit a shallower, broader style. Large-framed ladies: be mindful of wearing busy geometric patterns as they will only serve to enlarge your proportions. Try instead to accentuate your waist by wearing a belt with a decorative buckle and ensure that your dress or skirt stops at the slimmest part of your leg.

MEN'S LOOK

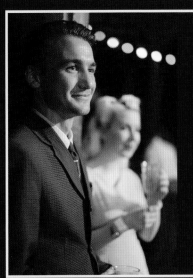

Personal grooming is a must: for even though a gentleman's hair may be hidden under a hat, it is imperative that it is slick and groomed. so it's worth keeping a small comb in your inside pocket. This same principle should apply to your moustache of choice, which should be combed, waxed, twirled at the ends and turned slightly upwards for that fashionable thirties finish. Don't forget about your hands and nails, too. Invest in some hand cream and keep your nails short and clean at all times.

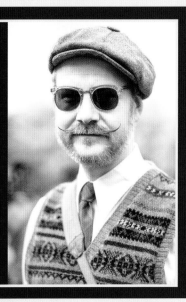

COOL CREAMS

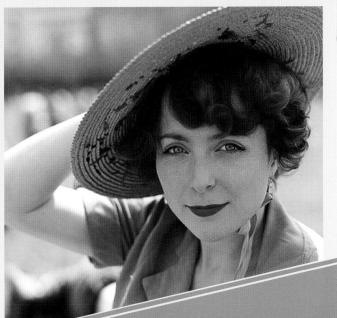

Make-up remained more natural than in the previous decade and this was also true of skin tones. Keep complexions fresh and clear by using Boots traditional cold-cream cleansers and toners that come in great retro packaging and be sure to invest in a pot of Elizabeth Arden's Eight Hour Cream, which made its cosmetic debut in the thirties and is a great alternative to Vaseline.

HEAVEN SCENT

By the 1930s. fragrances had become popular for both sexes. Women's perfume typically had light floral or oriental tones like jasmine, while men's aftershaves had mossy, woody scents with strong musk undertones. One of the most exciting perfumes of this period was Guerlain's *Djedi* a heady, spicy and smoky perfume, presented in a Hermès leather box with gold lamé lining. Some popular thirties fragrances are still worn today so. look out for; *Tabu* (House of Dana, 1932). *Je Reviens* (House of Worth, 1932), *Vol De Nuit* (Guerlain, 1933). *Blue Grass* (Elizabeth Arden, 1934), *Kobako* (Bourjois, 1936), *Angélique Encens* (Creed. 1933), and not forgetting *Dunhill for Men* (1934).

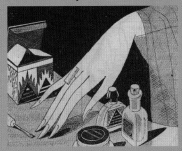

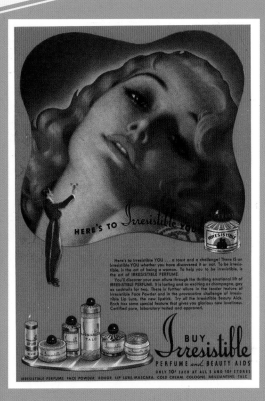

ASK THE EXPERT

Buttons

The Button Queen is a specialist shop in London that has been trading for over 60 years. Now run by Martyn and Isabel Frith, it was founded by Martyn's mother, Toni, who was an antique dealer in the 1950s.

What types of materials are vintage buttons made from?

You name a material and there have been buttons made from it! That's the beauty of buttons; there is no hard and fast rule. Looking back over history you will find buttons in brass, silver, gold, wood, Bakelite, plastic and, particularly during the world wars, buttons were made from glass as there was a shortage of other materials.

The Button Queen shop in London has thousands of buttons spanning many decades and styles.

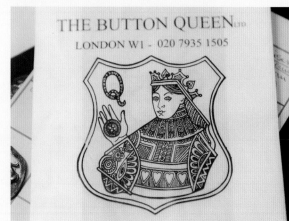

If someone is thinking about collecting buttons, where's a good place to start?

At home! Ask older members of the family. In the past, nothing was thrown away. If clothes started to become worn, they would simply be altered and only when they had completely perished were they cut up and used for dusters. Buttons would always be cut away and put into a tin to be reused. Go through the tins and pick out the ones you like. Talk to members of the family to ask if they remember where the buttons came from or what kind of clothes they were on.

Where else could you search for vintage buttons?

A lot of charity shops won't take buttons as it's too labour intensive to clean and put them on button cards to sell. But look out for old vintage clothes in charity shops that might have buttons that you can use on other garments. Try junk shops, antique shops and auctions, garage sales and car-boot sales for jars of buttons or clothes that have old buttons on them.

Are buttons from different eras easily recognizable and what are the details to look for?

Button shapes and decoration will often reflect the period in which they were made so it can be easy to identify an era. Buttons were mostly machine made from the twenties onwards so there tends to be more precision and uniformity in decoration. There were a lot of plastic buttons in the Art Deco style of the twenties and thirties. Due to the restriction on materials during World War II, many buttons made in the forties were from glass. Hand-painted and themed buttons were big in the fifties and sixties, whilst in the seventies buttons were made from metal or wood. The eighties saw a lot of metal and enamel buttons, and in the nineties, plastic and ceramic ones were often used. But there was also a trend for Chinese and Japanese buttons which were made from carved peach stones.

These grand and sophisticated buttons are a contrast to some of the more fun buttons available, such as the swan and top hat on the opposite page.

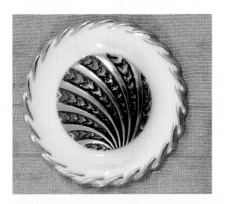

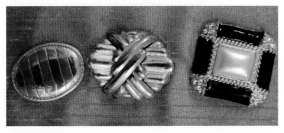

What type of buttons are good to collect?

Buttons can be made from precious metals, which will have a scrap value as well as an aesthetic one. Designer buttons are very collectable, too, especially labels like Chanel, Westood and Dior. Again, look in charity shops or clothes shops that have second-hand designer wear. Military buttons from major wars, and buttons from celebrity clothing and film costumes will also be valuable but you should be able to verify the provenance.

Choose a colour, choose an era, choose a shape... whatever your choice, a generic theme is a great way to start a button collection... or several!

What sort of collection should someone start?

Collect buttons that have a special meaning for you, such as a type that reminds you of your childhood, or from your favourite vintage era. You could start a themed collection just because you like a certain colour or shape or animal. Here are some other suggestions to give you inspiration:

* Brass buttons
* Glass buttons from the Victorian era
* Bohemian glass
* Celluloid (early plastic) buttons popular from the 1900s to 1920s
* Bakelite buttons popular in the USA from the 1920s to 1940s
* Evening-wear buttons
* Fabric-covered buttons

Browsing through trays of buttons will give you inspiration, and most shop owners are happy to talk about their passion.

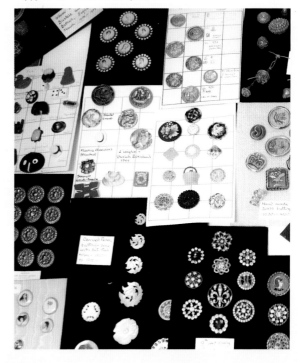

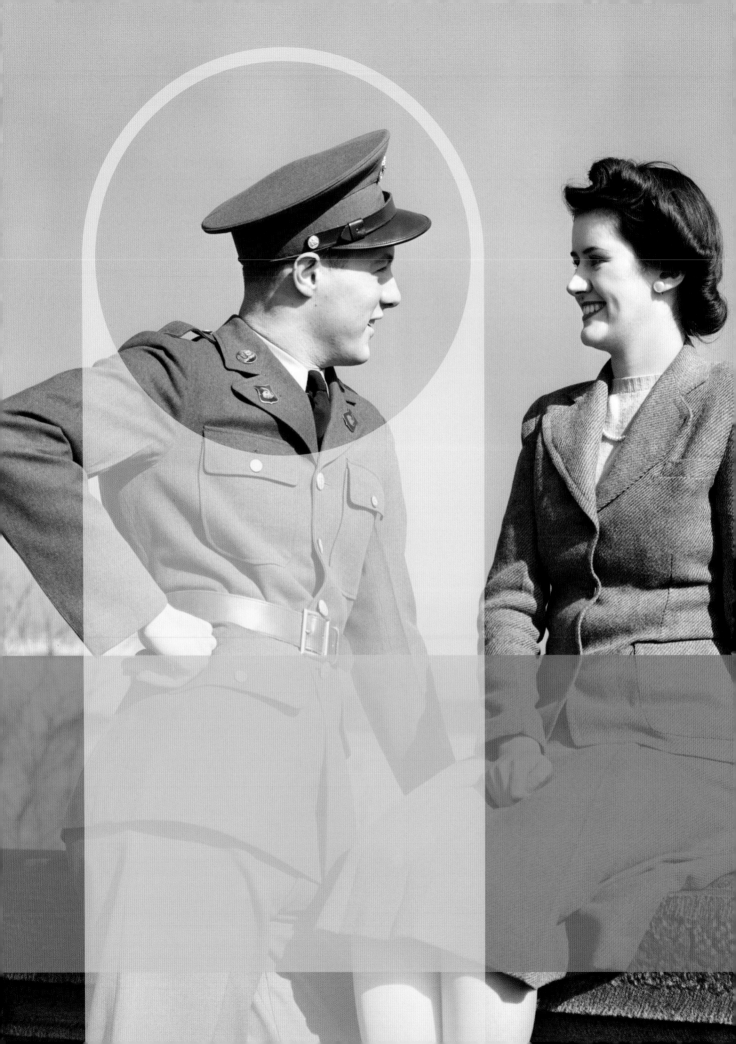

1940s

The 1940s were dominated by World War II and were synonymous with struggle and hardship. The German army marched into Paris in June 1940 and took control and, as the first year of the new decade came to an end, the City of London was devastated by heavy German bombing, which came to be known as the Blitz. However, the British government and many companies were keen to remain positive and promoted a 'business as usual' attitude. As a result, despite many shortages and problems of supply, the British fashion industry carried on regardless.

London, Paris and Milan, the cities that made major contributions to clothing manufacture and haute couture, were all to experience change on an overwhelming scale. Dyes, fabrics, plastics and metals were diverted to the war effort and so the early years of 1940s fashion were shrouded in bleakness. However, the fashion industry did not grind to a complete halt. Those individuals with the means to barter were able to obtain 'black market' goods, especially as rationing was not imposed as heavily in certain countries or all at the same time. Some of the top fashion houses even managed to present small collections and do as much business during the war as they had before.

Clothes rationing was introduced in Britain in June 1941, and by the end of the year the British Board of Trade was advising housewives to 'Make Do and Mend', issuing brochures offering advice on how this could be achieved. With stoic resolve and invention, many people found ways to cling on to a degree of fashion consciousness throughout the decade. Sewing became a necessary skill to ensure that what little they had could be maintained and repaired. With a substantial percentage of the world's population wearing a military uniform of some description for the first half of the decade, a flurry of designs for ladies' military-cut suits emerged, together with the siren suit, modelled on workmen's overalls, and so called because they were all-in-one outfits that could be quickly slipped over pyjamas when the night-time air raid siren was heard. They became a fashion statement for the rich and famous, who wore them over their evening clothes if there was a raid.

Following the introduction of 'utility clothing' in 1941, the British Government commissioned some of the most esteemed designers of the day: Hardy Amies, Bianca Mosca, Edward Molyneux, Digby Morton, Norman Hartnell and Victor Stiebel, to create durable wardrobe essentials for both men and women. They produced 34 designs for the Civilian Clothing range of 1941, or CC41 as it was called, which included streamlined and stylish dresses; which proved popular, although choice was understandably limited. The patriotic colours of 'war wise' clothing included air-force blue, flag red, black, brown, green and grey flannel.

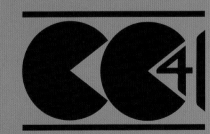

1940s WOMEN'S DAY WEAR

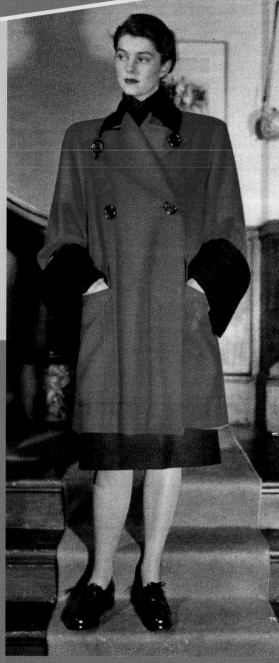

During the war years raw materials, such as cloth, wool and leather, were in short supply and most factories changed their output to focus on the war effort. Wool, for example, was used for service uniforms. The utility clothing ranges that were introduced used the minimum amount of fabric and were simple and plain in design. No turn-ups for trousers were allowed and no fastenings, such as press studs and zips, were permitted. There were also limits on the number of pleats, buttons and pockets. But women still wanted to look good, so many mended or picked apart the contents of their wardrobes and unravelled or reused garments for the family; non-rationed blackout cloth was even revamped into trousers and lingerie. As the war continued, the clothing coupon allowance was cut and many families were too poor to buy new clothes.

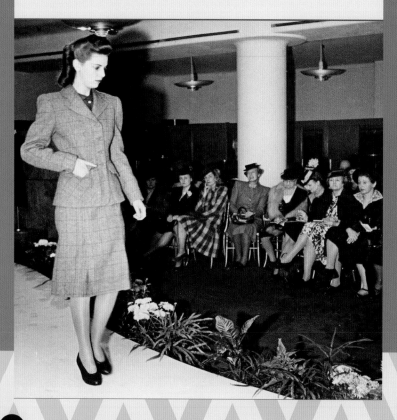

The post-war years did not bring an immediate change to either the style or accessibility of fashion, but the demand for chic never waned. The most notable difference after 1945 was the increase in the amount of material available for women's outer-wear. This created a much squarer and broader shoulder to the silhouette. The use of patriotic red was popular, together with both white and blue. Styles appeared with double breasting and oversize cuffs and buttons, which would have been considered far too extravagant only a few years before.

MATERIAL GIRL

Although fashion in its truest form still existed during the war, prints and patterns were only accessible to the very wealthy who could afford to pay the right people to source fabrics that were increasingly hard to get hold of. Many fabrics featured patriotic or propaganda motifs, but these were more common in the United States, where rationing was not as stringent. In Britain, the Women's Land Army re-formed, and volunteers, known as Land Girls, wore heavy-duty dungarees, known as bib and brace overalls, which the girls tried to make sexy by cinching in at the waist. After the war, long dungaree-style culottes caught on as casual wear, together with variations of the one-piece siren suit, which were adapted into short, flirty play suits. Skirt hems dropped below the knee and the volume of material increased, making longer skirts and dresses perfect for the new styles of dances, such as the Lindy Hop and Jitterbug.

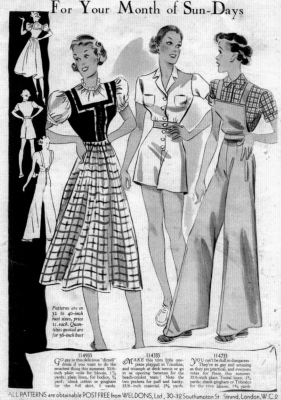

For Your Month of Sun-Days

Thousands of women, behind the men, behind the guns, working in factories had to keep practicality and clothing coupons at the front of their minds when buying clothes. Irish fashion designer Digby Morton created what was to become the perfect uniform for factory workers, cleverly made in three pieces, which could be replaced separately at two coupons for trousers or top, and one for the detachable apron. It was government sponsored and available in most factories, which allowed women to continue to look their best at all times without veering outside the confines of rationing.

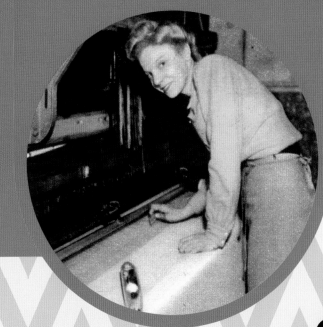

WAISTED!

Rationing required blouses to have a plain design with only a simple breast pocket permitted. This meant that many early styles were made for functionality rather than form. However, as the 1940s drew to an end, new designs were constructed from gossamer materials with a particular emphasis on bows, which gave women's clothes a delicate and feminine feel. Raglan and dolman sleeves with bulky shoulder pads dominated and were teamed with knee-length skirt suits. Callot Soeurs Ltd and Jaques Fath produced high-quality women's clothing, with their designs showing off a nipped-in waist, which started a trend that would last well into the next decade.

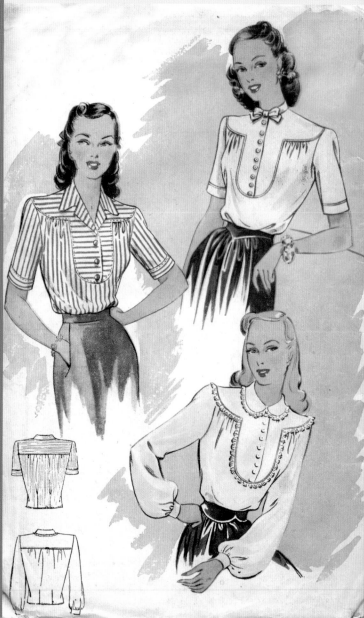

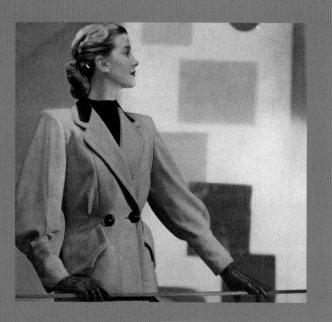

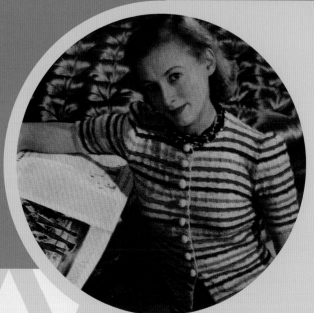

KNITTING PRETTY

Wool was in short supply throughout the forties with production diverted to where it was needed most – the war effort. Materials such as jersey wool, rayon and crepe were used as alternatives, with existing knitwear unpicked and re-fashioned into new pieces. The styles of the early decade favoured a simple round neck, while the post-war years saw ladies' décolletage exposed with V-neck and scoop-neck designs. Sleeve length varied according to the practicality of the piece, with a few individuals creating faux jumpers that consisted of a knitted front panel with back ties that created the illusion of a complete garment. Knitting patterns could be found everywhere, including in periodicals and magazines, although continental knitting became unpopular due to its Germanic heritage.

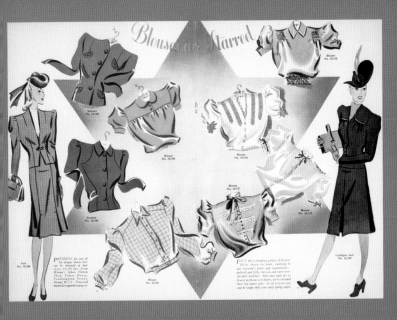

Blouses are Starred

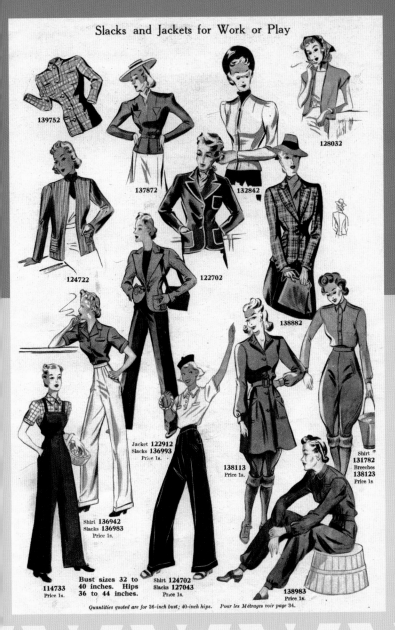

Slacks and Jackets for Work or Play

139752

128032

137872

132842

124722

122702

138882

Jacket 122912
Slacks 136993
Price 1s.

138113
Price 1s.

Shirt
131782
Breeches
138123
Price 1s

Shirt 136942
Slacks 136983
Price 1s.

Shirt 124702
Slacks 127043
Price 1s.

114733
Price 1s.

Bust sizes 32 to
40 inches. Hips
36 to 44 inches.

138983
Price 1s.

Quantities quoted are for 36-inch bust; 40-inch hips.   Pour les Métrages voir page 34.

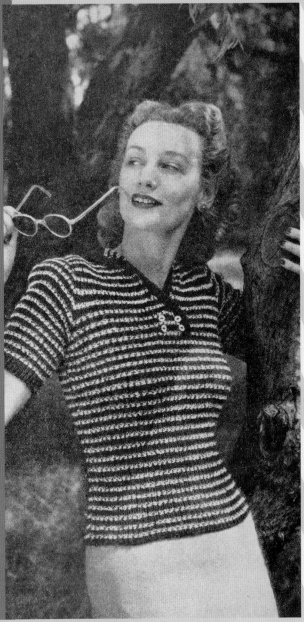

SEPARATE SOLUTIONS

During the forties, women were called upon to fulfil roles previously only considered for men, giving rise to a demand for functional yet feminine outfits that would double for work and play. As a result of rationing, the concept of separates really took off – women needed to get the most out of their wardrobe for as long as possible. Having 'classic' pieces of clothing that could be mixed and matched allowed wearers to create the illusion of variety, helped by the use of accessories, such as costume jewellery, hats, scarves, gloves and belts. This gave women the opportunity to create a sense of unique style and was a catalyst for some of the design concepts that followed.

940s MEN'S DAY WEAR

If you weren't fighting in the war, the correct etiquette for men was to appear as austere as possible. The average man's wardrobe consisted of a white shirt, rayon tie, woollen pullover, slim-leg pleated-front trousers and a pair of brogue shoes. Socks were navy, black, grey or brown and all men owned a hat. Undershirts or vests were a luxury but, if available, came from manufacturers such as Henleys. The rivalry between American GIs and home-grown soldiers extended into fashion throughout the war years and beyond, with the many Hollywood films portraying colourful fashion in stark contrast to the neutral tones seen in Britain at the time. The basic slim-fit, single-breasted suit had three buttons without pocket flaps or turn-ups. The lounge suit was also single breasted but was worn with two front buttons.

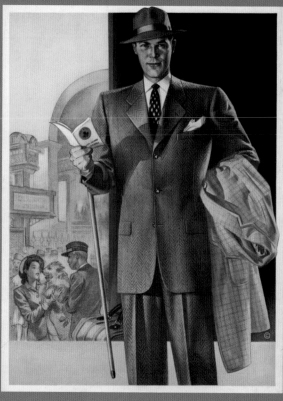

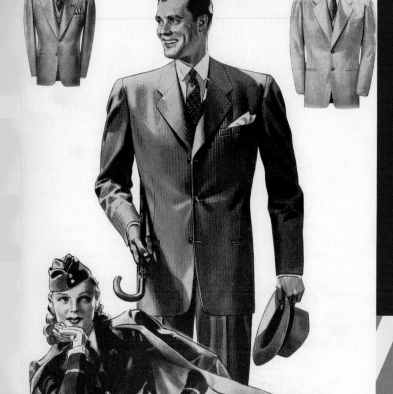

The style of men's overcoats was mainly double breasted with excessively broad shoulders, wide-notch lapels and perhaps one or two flap pockets. Some versions were belted.

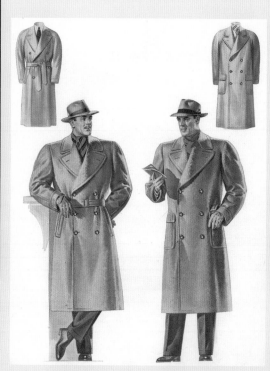

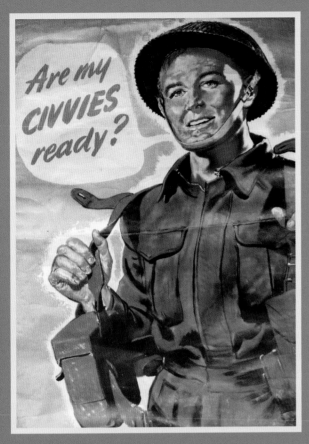

DEMOB HAPPY

At the end of the war, British men were demobilized from the armed forces. Having spent years in military uniform, their civilian wardrobes had meanwhile become casualties of war, so the government funded a civilian clothing programme.. The men received a trilby-style felt hat or optional flat cap; a double-breasted pinstripe three-piece suit, or a single-breasted jacket with flannel trousers; two shirts with matching collar studs; a tie; shoes and a raincoat. While the suits were made from good-quality fabric, they weren't made to measure and could be extremely ill-fitting. As a result, demob suits were often the subject of ridicule.

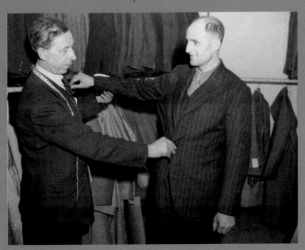

Get the Look with Hannah

Burberry, Simpsons and Austin Reed were reputable names in high-street fashion during the 1940s. Purchasing an original, well-tailored, correctly fitting overcoat, either single or double breasted, in a quality material such as Harris Tweed, cashmere or Venetian wool, is an investment. These styles are timeless but it is important to check for damage and to be aware of the appropriate storage options to keep the coat in great condition. If your wallet permits, consider having a coat made to measure using modern fabrics and team this with a time-honoured fedora hat for the quintessential forties debonair look.

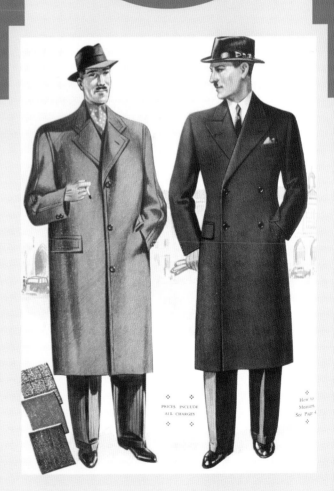

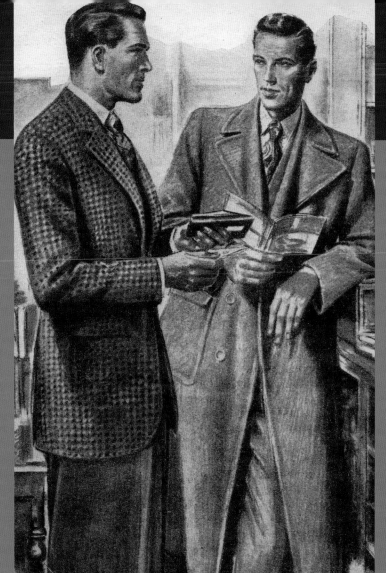

TIE-INS

Hand-painted silk ties were all the rage in the late forties, from the elegant to the exotic and, in some cases, the risqué. Considered exhibitionist by the more modest British male, the concept of the 'Bold Look' evolved in America, where returning servicemen sought relief from the repression of war and a more stimulating colour palette, reminiscent of the twenties and early thirties. Many ties were designed with geometric patterns and were worn with everyday suits. However, as the trend caught on, more elaborate and themed artwork was displayed. Peek-a-boo ties hid their true nature; usually incredibly plain to the naked eye, when flipped over and gently parted they revealed a sexy pin-up girl, similar to the fighter-plane nose art that was popular during the war.

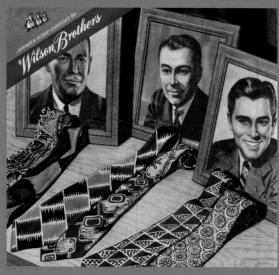

CHARITY SHOP

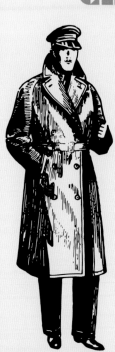

The aftermath of World War II saw many men return to very little and some to nothing. Homes, families and workplaces had been ravaged by the conflict, resulting in dire poverty for many, long after peace was declared. And so the charity shop was born. Although the practise of donating used items to a charity to raise money was not unheard of, permanent shops were uncommon. However, during the 1940s, over 350 outlets were set up by the Red Cross to support those in need, with the vast majority of donations being made up of the clothes and personal effects of fallen heroes. The 'waste not, want not' attitude was maintained and resulted in many of the styles and outfits from the pre-war years resurfacing later in the decade, even though wearing 'vintage' was an unknown fashion concept at the time.

Get the Look with Hannah

Smelling 'manly' by wearing a fragrance was still a novel concept during the forties but was fast becoming popular down to some clever marketing. Splash on a little *Old Spice* for an authentic retro aroma.

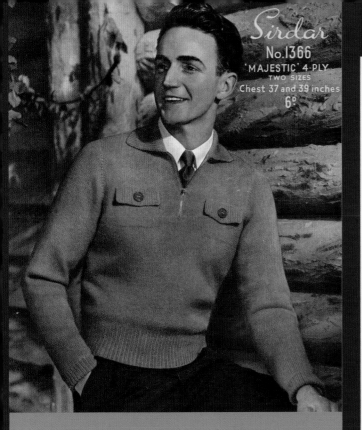

MEN'S KNITWEAR

Men's knitwear became more plentiful during the late forties, and with Europe experiencing one of the worst winters on record in 1946-47, there was never a better time to own a woolly jumper. The V neckline was the most popular style. However, natural yarns were still difficult or expensive to obtain so knitting or buying a new jumper was a costly option. As a result, a lot of old knitwear was unpicked and the yarn reused. Knitted waistcoats were a great way to layer up and became something of a fashion statement. Plain colours in knitted waistcoats were less popular than bolder or geometric designs and would be worn with a white shirt and tie.

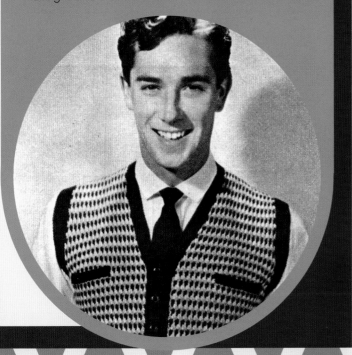

Reliable Outfit

Big Yank was a subsidiary brand of the Reliance Manufacturing Company founded in Chicago in 1919, and its utilitarian clothing was in demand in the forties. In 1942, the company patented the term 'convenient pocket' on the left side of its shirts and jackets. These pyramid-shaped pockets were known as sweat-proof pockets and were used to hold cigarettes, fob watches and other items that had to be kept dry and perspiration free. Other features of the brand were 'storm cuffs', which were made without a placket so that the wearer could avoid getting caught in machinery, and a strain-proof yoke for ease of movement.

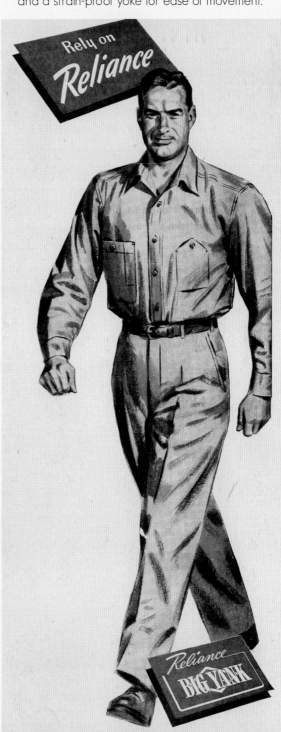

Rely on *Reliance*

Reliance BIG YANK

1940s WOMEN'S EVENING WEAR

Throughout the war years people were still keen to have fun and many flocked to the decadent nightclubs that had sprung up in the twenties and thirties. Bars in deep underground locations thrived, where men and women listened and danced to loud swing music, which helped to drown out the air-raid sirens above. Everyone sought to escape the monotony and horror of war, and also defiantly to maintain the 'Keep Calm and Carry On', motto coined at the start of the war. Glamour was well represented in the 1940s and, with the advent of Christian Dior's New Look collection in 1947, was to become synonymous with the golden age of Hollywood films. Movie-star goddesses like Rita Hayworth, as seen in the 1946 film *Gilda* (below), were promoted as 'Glamour Girls' with long, wavy hairstyles, revealing dresses and a devil-may-care attitude. Cinched waists and the revival of the décolletage focused women on exercise in order to keep a slim body shape.

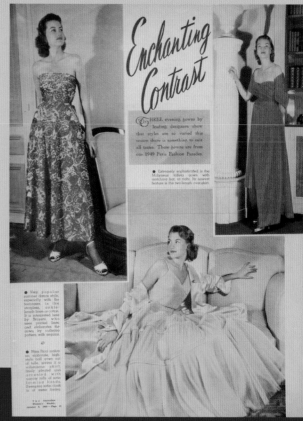

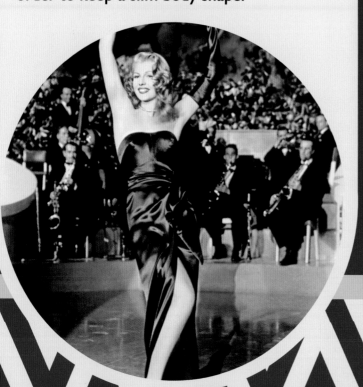

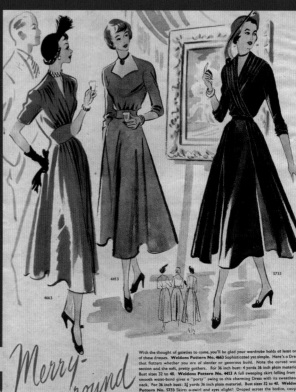

BORROWED FROM THE BOYS!

Bolero jackets were another feature of late forties evening wear. First noted on Spanish men in the early nineteenth century, they were a later influence on the design of jackets worn by Victorian ladies. Finishing just above the waist, the bolero was the perfect style to accentuate the nipped-in waist that was being emphasized in fashion magazines such as *Vogue*.

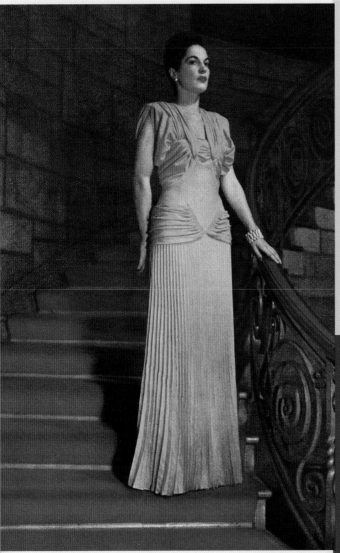

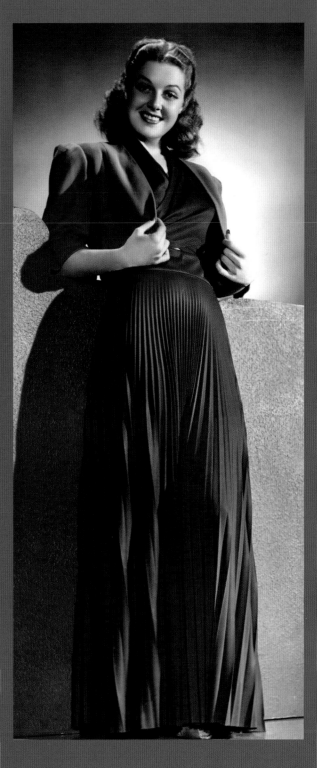

PLEATS PLEASE

When France was liberated in 1944, Parisian couture was reinstated as the height of chic. In the post-war period, the female silhouette was beginning to alter. The greatest fashion changes were seen in the new sleeve styles and, with thick shoulder pads making an entrance in the late forties, the head of the sleeve would typically be darted or gathered. Pleating and gathering of fabrics became desirable too, as designers were now able to use more material to create stitchbox or knife pleats in dresses and skirts, helping to create softer lines and a less uniform feel to fashion.

THE NEW LOOK

In 1947, a Reuters correspondent dubbed fashion designer Christian Dior's latest collection the 'New Look'. Dior wanted to return to women a light-heartedness as well as the power of seduction in their dress. He wanted cutting patterns that emphasized the bust and waist, and allowed freedom of movement (see below). Somewhat ironically, the diminutive waistlines could only be achieved using a guêpière – a type of corset – which when positioned just above the yards of gathered percale and taffeta created a visually stunning contrast to anything seen in recent years. Dior's New Look collection featured shirring, dolman sleeves and rounded shoulders, which were a contrast to the style of the early decade which popularized a broad, square frame using shoulder pads. Stiff high collars and deep V necklines helped create the perfect hourglass shape representative of his favourite number, eight.

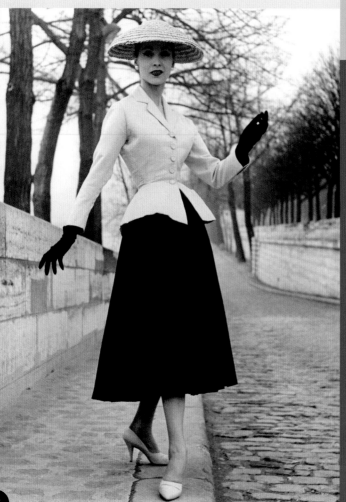

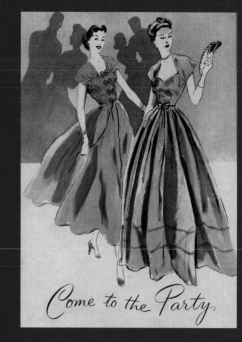

Come to the Party

CLEVER DETAIL

Decorative embellishment was a big feature of women's evening wear, with sequins and beads simulating jewels. This characteristic detailing allowed women of the forties to add a touch of sparkle to their otherwise simple attire, which was still restricted by clothes rationing. Appliqué and piqué appliqué could be found on plainer evening wear, and lace was often used over the fabric of the bodice to create texture and detail. Silk and moiré sashes were a feature on tulle gowns, as were oversize back bows. However, these decorative features only appeared after the war when it became acceptable once more to use extra fabric to accessorize garments.

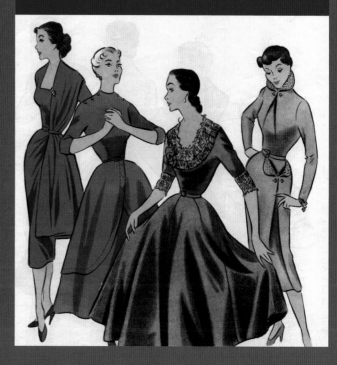

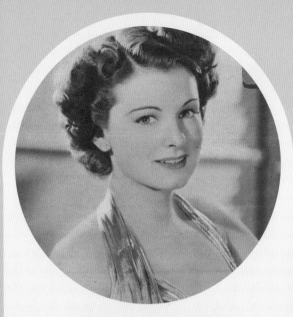

EXPOSURE

As dress designers sampled new ideas, necklines on evening wear started to expose the neck, back and décolletage. This required both the inner structure of the garment and the lingerie to support the wearer. As a result, great focus was placed on the design and practicality of underwear.

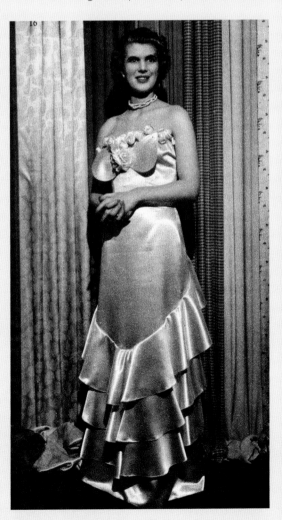

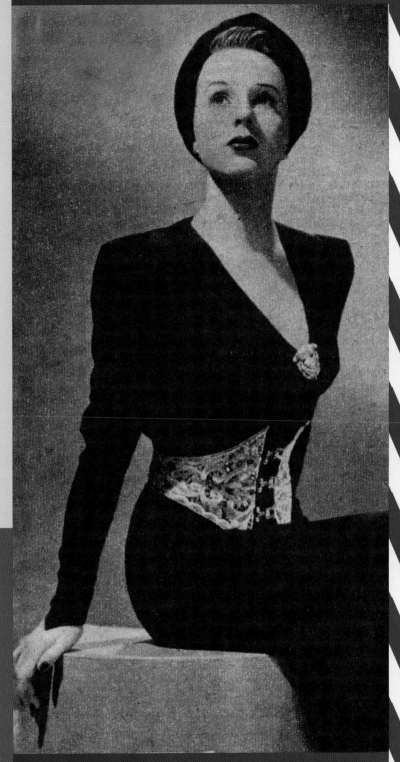

CAGED IN

The dimensions of the female waist became such a focus in the late forties that it wasn't long before hand-span belts became all the rage. A 'waist cincher' could be worn over your stays to further minimize the skeletal void between your ribs and your Ilium but still remain underneath your evening gown. 'Cage belts', like the one worn by Hollywood actress Deanna Durbin above, could also be worn over your ensemble as designs became more intricate and bejewelled. However, they weren't always the most comfortable item and required the wearer to maintain an upright posture at all times!

Full evening dress changed after the war and white tie and tails were considered apropriate for only the most formal of functions. Semi-formal dinner jackets or tuxedos appealed to a broader audience, particularly in the United States where the 'Bold Look' was launched by *Apparel Arts* and *Esquire* magazines in the late 1940s, embracing brash, broad lapels and wide-pleat shirts. The 'Mr T' (Mr Trim) look was a much more reticent silhouette with streamlined characteristics. In warmer climes, white single- or double-breasted shawl collars were permitted and post-war etiquette continued to allow colour in accessories, although they were now generally limited to subdued black, midnight blue or maroon.

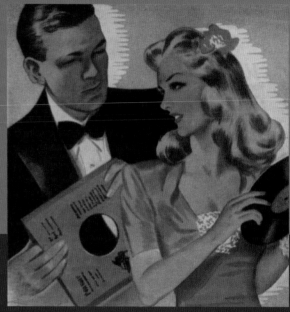

BOW TIES

Choosing the most appropriate bow tie model separated the gentleman from the waiter and, much like today, it was regarded as incongruous to wear a pre-tied bow tie to a formal function. Colour was almost always black, although midnight-blue was an acceptable alternative. Patterned and multicoloured varieties were avoided at all costs. Shape, however, was imperative, with classic and modern butterfly shapes differing in size by up to one inch.

CORRECT MODELS FOR FORMAL ATTIRE

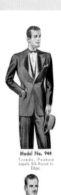

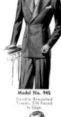

Model No. 944 — Tuxedo. Peaked Lapels. Silk Faced to Edge.
V-320 — Single-Breasted Dress Vest with rounded collar.
V-321 — Single-Breasted Dress Vest with square collar.
V-322 — Double-Breasted Dress Vest with collar.
Back of 944, 945, 946, 947, 949 and 950. No vent.
Model No. 945 — Double-Breasted Tuxedo. Silk Faced to Edge.

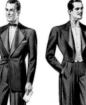
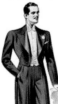
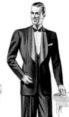
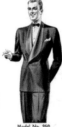

Model No. 946 — Double-Breasted Tuxedo. Piped Pockets. Silk Faced to Edge.
Model No. 947 — Tuxedo. Notch Lapels. Silk Faced to Edge.
Model No. 948 — Full Dress for Formal Evening Wear. Peaked Lapels. Silk Faced to Edge.
Model No. 949 — Shawl Collar Tuxedo. Piped Pockets. Silk Faced to Edge.
Model No. 950 — Double-Breasted Shawl Collar Tuxedo. Piped Pockets. Silk Faced to Edge.

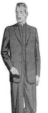
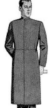
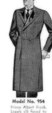

Model No. 951 — Drop-Button Clerical Sack. Notch Lapels.
Model No. 952 — Clerical Frock. When ordering give size of linen collar worn.
Model V-323 — Clerical Vest. When ordering give size of linen collar worn.
V-324 — Cassock Vest. When ordering give size of linen collar worn.
Model No. 953 — One-Button Cutaway Frock. Peaked Lapels.
Model No. 956 — Prince Albert Frock. Lapels silk Faced to buttonholes.

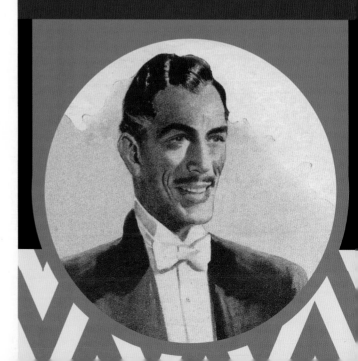

ZOOT SUIT REBELS

At no time considered suitable attire by discerning gentlemen, Zoot Suits were regarded as exhibitionist and chichi. Associated with rebellion, these suits were sported by those frequenting 'unsavoury' nightclubs and were considered hugely unpatriotic because of the large amounts of material needed to make them. Lacking structure, the trousers had a high waist and low crotch, with extensive room around the rear and thighs, and the legs tapering dramatically to the ankle. Jackets were equally excessive in drape, with padded, broad shoulders and wide lapels. The length of a jacket typically fell to the mid-thigh. The cut of the 'Zoot' meant there was more allowance for different body shapes. Materials varied according to affordability or occasion. Wool was the most expensive and therefore the most sought after material for a Zoot.

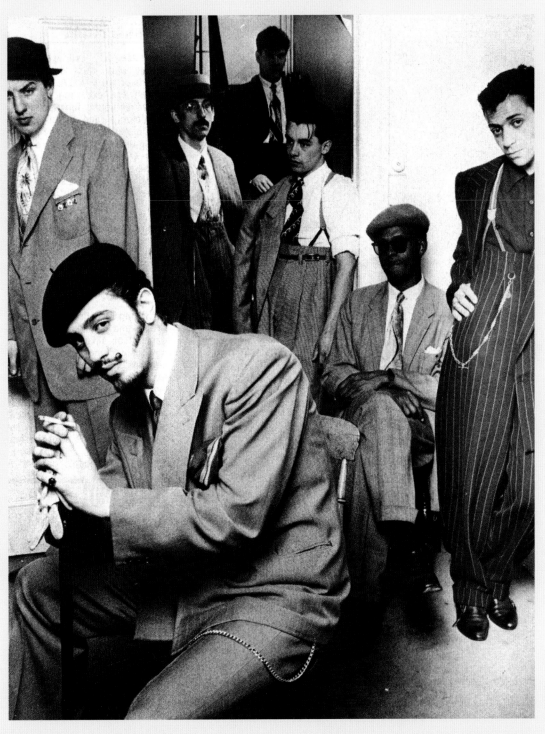

1940s SHOES

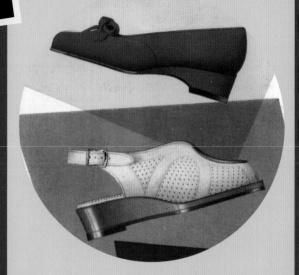

Shoe manufacturing had become a far less labour-intensive process by the 1940s. The delicate dance shoes of the previous two decades gracefully tiptoed into the shadows as World War II advanced, and were replaced mainly by practical day-to-evening alternatives like court shoes. Established shoe manufacturers, such as Clarks, ran widely successful campaigns advertising their range of hinged wooden shoes whilst the Airborne Company offered a range for teens, recognizable today as the company behind the Kickers brand.

IF THE SHOE FITS

Women's shoes underwent a radical change in design at both the beginning and end of the decade. The increasing heel height of ladies' shoes was halted for several years while attention in technology was diverted to the war. Alternatives to leather bases were created with the use of wood and cork. The wedge, despite using more base material than regular shoes, offered greater height, longevity and sturdiness. It was also regarded as being far more 'fashionable' and became a design that has remained popular to the present day. After the war shoes became less utilitarian and more decorative.

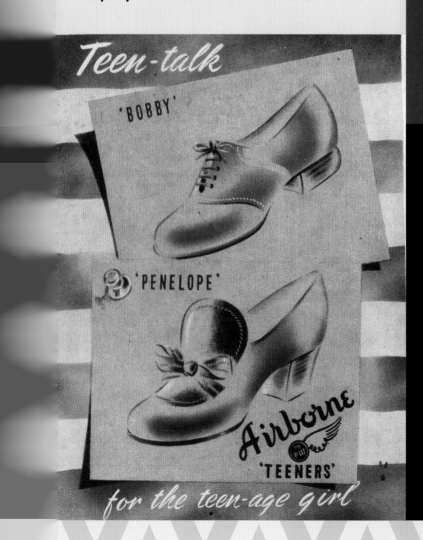

Teen-talk

'BOBBY'

'PENELOPE'

Airborne

'TEENERS'

for the teen-age girl

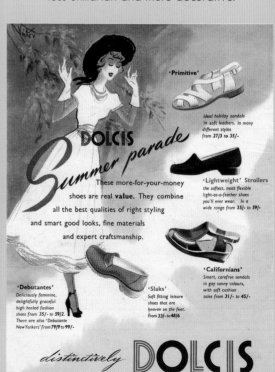

DOLCIS

Summer parade

These more-for-your-money shoes are real **value**. They combine all the best qualities of right styling and smart good looks, fine materials and expert craftsmanship.

'Primitive'
Ideal holiday sandals in soft leathers. In many different styles from 27/3 to 35/-.

'Lightweight' Strollers the softest, most flexible light-as-a-feather shoes you'll ever wear. In a wide range from 35/- to 59/-

'Californians' Smart, carefree sandals in gay sunny colours, with soft cushion soles from 31/- to 45/-

'Debutantes' Deliciously feminine, delightfully graceful high heeled fashion shoes from 35/- to 59/2. There are also 'Debutante New Yorkers' from 79/9 to 99/-

'Slaks' Soft fitting leisure shoes that are heaven on the feet. From 33/- to 48/6

distinctively DOLCIS

CLASSIC SHOES

The majority of women's shoes tended to have a rounded toe with a more robust block, lavatory or Louis heel. Court shoes remained a classic style and were embellished with accessories. Names such as Salvatore Ferragamo, Roger Vivier and Russell and Bromley designed collections for the affluent shopper of the time, while more affordable labels, such as Lilley & Skinner, Norvic and Dolcis, served those of moderate means.

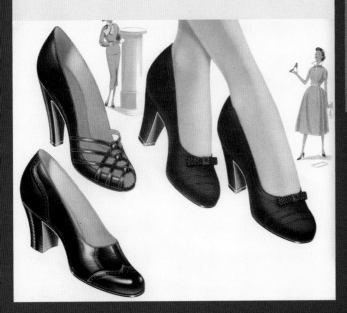

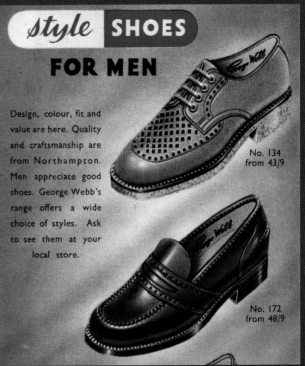
For men, Oxford brogues remained the favoured design choice, together with saddle shoes or, for the more relaxed, the loafer. Modern manufacturing took into account the necessity for dual-purpose use, by providing thicker soles and heels that were suitable for both work and play. Formality was essential for both day and evening wear, which meant a preference for laces over slip-ons. The discerning gent went to shoemakers, such as Tricker's, for hand-made bespoke footwear, a company that is still flourishing today.

MARCHING BOOTS

Most raw materials during the first half of the decade were used to support the war effort, and leather for boots and shoes was no exception. As a result, leather became extremely expensive and most men had to make do with the shoes they had. After the war, many men with outdoor or factory jobs continued to wear their army boots as these were tough and hard-wearing. However, designs such as half boots and ankle boots became popular with some working men, while patent leather varieties were available for businessmen.

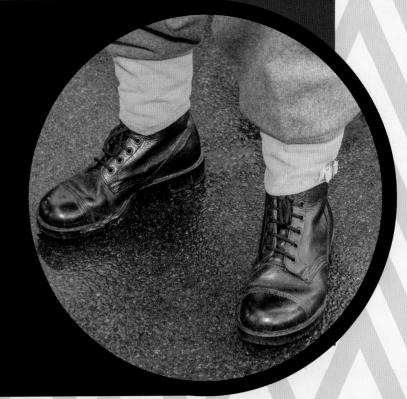

1940s SPORTSWEAR

Sport and sporting events around the world were seriously disrupted or more often cancelled as a result of the war. But football matches organized by the armed forces continued and were a way of keeping home-based servicemen fit and entertained. In the post-war years, the summer and winter Olympic Games returned as well as championship tennis at Wimbledon (below) and professional cricket (both 1946) and football (1945). However, sports clothing was still rather basic in the UK and much of it was reused from before 1939. America meanwhile had excelled in the production of sports and leisure clothing as rationing there was not as stringent as in the UK.

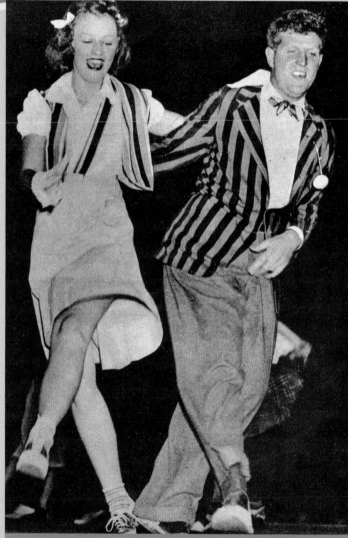

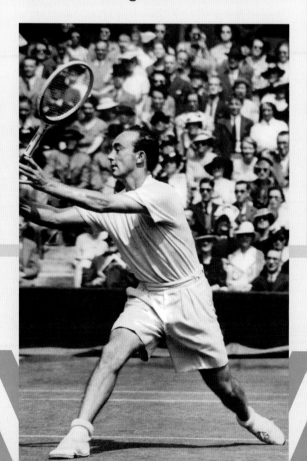

STEP LIVELY!

The big-band music of the early to mid-1940s, combined with human resilience and determination to carry on regardless, saw exercise, in the form of energetic dancing, pursued on a grand scale. Swing was embraced on both sides of the Atlantic and its frenetic dance moves required a new approach to leisure-wear design and materials.

America created its own look at this time, with designers producing mix and match sweaters worn over polo shirts, and button-down shirts and jackets to be worn with slacks. These made the perfect outfits for the fervid dance floor and could expand into leisure clothing designs for the future.

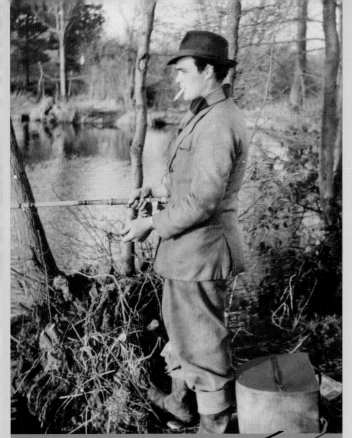

JACKETS

Astride the latest AJS 7R 'boy racer', casting your new nylon fishing line or swinging a cricket bat, the need to unwind and make the most of leisure time was never more important than in the forties. Sought-after pieces include Admiral Byrd horsehide leather jackets and items from the oldest British motorcycle company, Lewis Leathers. The latter were for fashion as well as racing. Based in London, the company still manufactures from original vintage designs using D Lewis, Lewis Leathers and Aviakit trademark labels.

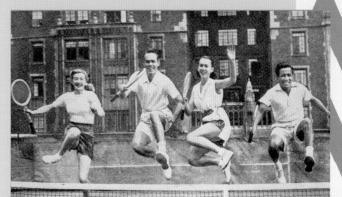

AUSTERITY GAMES

After a twelve-year suspension, the 1948 Summer Olympics were a breath of fresh air. Although the weather was some of the worst on record in the UK, the event held at London's Wembley Stadium was the first Olympics to be broadcast on television. Dubbed the 'austerity games', athletes struggled to get even the most basic clothing and footwear. British male competitors were supplied with two pairs of Y-fronts, a blazer and white trousers from Simpson's of Piccadilly, while the women were dressed by Bourne & Hollingsworth, a quality department store based in Oxford Street.

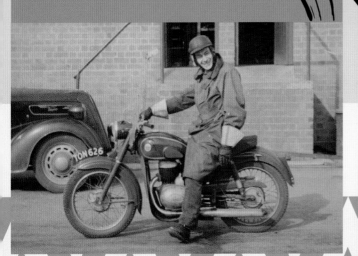

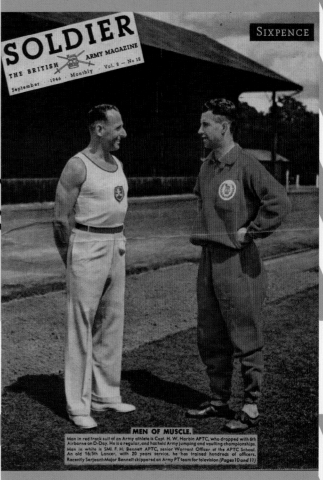

MEN OF MUSCLE.
Man in red track suit of an Army athlete is Capt. H. W. Harbin APTC, who dropped with 6th Airborne on D-Day. He is a regular, and has held Army jumping and vaulting championships. Man in white is SMI F. H. Bennett APTC, senior Warrant Officer at the APTC School. An old 16/5th Lancer, with 20 years service, he has trained hundreds of officers. Recently Serjeant-Major Bennett skippered an Army PT team for television (Pages 10 and 11).

1940s ACCESSORIES

With so much of 1940s life dominated by the necessity to make do and mend, it is not surprising that many women (and men) became proficient at knitting, sewing and embroidery. A wide selection of accessories were uniquely embellished, although only basic, accessible materials could be used. Everything from hats and handbags, to scarves and plain CC41 clothes were decorated to make them more attractive and to give the wearer a sense of individuality and style. Men's accessories also became popular and were a way of injecting a little detail into otherwise plain clothes. This lead to a demand in belts and braces and, in particular, tie pins and cufflinks.

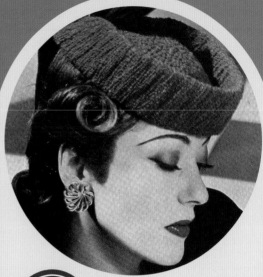

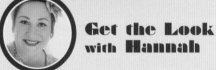

Get the Look with Hannah

Costume jewellery from the forties continued to mimic elaborate expensive designs. Named pieces are prized, so look out for Trifari, Eisenberg and Coro in particular. Gold tones were more popular than silver, and clip-on earrings were common. It is worth being aware that nickel was often used on cheap costume pieces, which can cause irritation to the skin. Rhinestones and crystal brooches are generally affordable and can be used in a variety of ways to accessorize coats, hats, bags scarves and jumpers. Fur clips have sharp prongs and, despite the name, are not designed to be worn with fur accessories as the clips would likely tear the fur. They are best suited to heavy materials on dresses or coats.

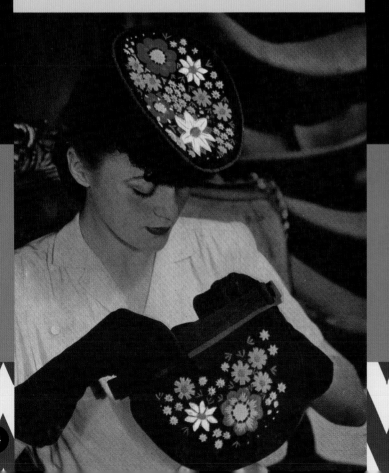

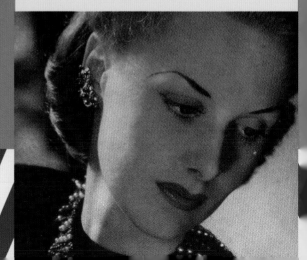

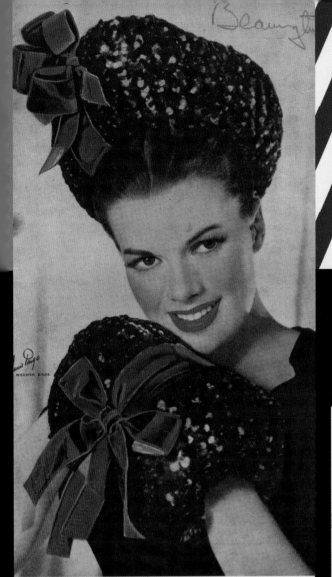

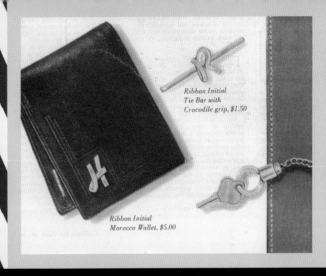

Ribbon Initial
Tie Bar with
Crocodile grip, $1.50

Ribbon Initial
Morocco Wallet, $5.00

MEN'S EXTRAS

Apart from colourful ties, most gentlemen's accessories remained traditional in colour and style. Leather gloves and fedora hats were a must, but if a man had items to carry he could choose a utility or travel bag or a simple 'handy' bag to complete his look.

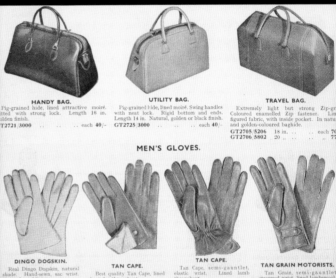

HANDY BAG.
Pig-grained hide, lined attractive moiré. Fitted with strong lock. Length 16 in. Golden finish.
GT2721/3000 .. .. each 40/-

UTILITY BAG.
Pig-grained hide, lined moiré. Swing handles with neat lock. Rigid bottom and ends. Length 14 in. Natural, golden or black finish.
GT2725/3000 .. .. each 40/-

TRAVEL BAG.
Extremely light but strong Zip-grip. Coloured enamelled Zip fastener. Lined figured fabric, with inside pocket. In natural and golden-coloured baghide.
GT2705/5206 18 in. .. .. each 70/-
GT2706/5802 20 .. .. 77/-

MEN'S GLOVES.

DINGO DOGSKIN.
Real Dingo Dogskin, natural shade. Hand-sewn, sac wrist. Knitted wool lining.
GC4870/1103 .. per pair 15/-

TAN CAPE.
Best quality Tan Cape, lined lawn fur throughout.
GC4872/1509 .. per pair 21/-

TAN CAPE.
Tan Cape, semi-gauntlet, elastic wrist. Lined lamb throughout.
GC4875/1500 .. per pair 20/-

TAN GRAIN MOTORISTS.
Tan Grain, semi-gauntlet strapped wrist, lined lambswool.
GC4878/1306 .. per pair 18/-

MAD HATTER

Many materials used by milliners were exempt from rationing, which gave them carte blanche when it came to creativity. Women's hat shapes included the pill-box (far left and top left), which was most usually a flat, cylindrical shape that sat close to the head; these were often teamed with bird-cage lace, feathers and flowers as well as bows, which were big during the decade. Turbans were made famous by Marlene Dietrich and came as ready-made, although many achieved the same look with a large scarf. Wearing a neck scarf was still quintessentially English and in the 1940s brands such as Liberty and Hermès were just as desirable as they are today.

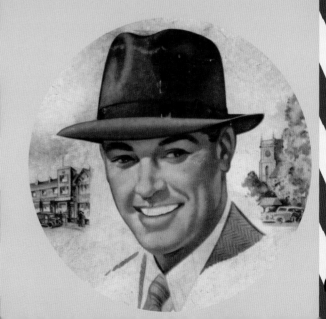

1940s GET THE LOOK WITH HANNAH

A good handbag is a simple and effective way to get the forties look without having to spend a fortune. The shape of a typical bag from this period is very distinctive. It won't be designed to be worn on the shoulder – instead it should be carried in the crook of the arm or as a clutch bag. It will be structured and will generally have a top clasp fastening. Referred to as a 'granny bag', it's worth asking older relatives if they have any examples lurking in a wardrobe. Otherwise, charity shops are a great place to look and will usually be relatively inexpensive compared to specialist vintage shops.

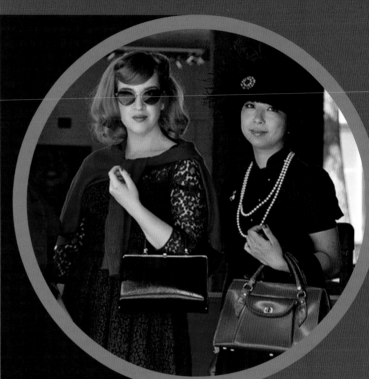

MAKE DO AND VINTAGE

Apply the make do and mend mentality from this decade and breathe a little fresh air back into tired items or simply re-create vintage style using modern materials. Don't dismiss hats that are marginally too tight or a bit flat from being squashed in a suitcase in the attic; get them stretched and steamed, and adorn them with feathers, flowers, ribbons or brooches for a quirky twist. Add vintage-style buttons to jackets or cardigans. Fat quarters of material can easily be turned into handkerchiefs for gentlemen, too, which make great presents and allow you to use leftover material from sewing projects.

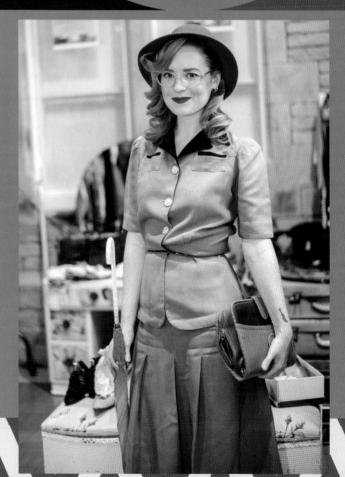

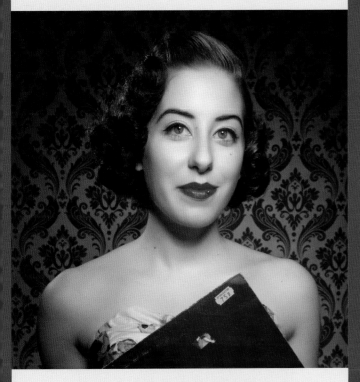

TIME FOR A VICTORY ROLL

The forties look is all about soft, curled hair, strong red lips and dramatic eyebrows. Pick a shade of red lipstick most suited to your skin tone for a fabulous forties pout. For brows, use a pencil or powder to fill in the gaps of your natural brows, making sure you shape them from thick at the inner edge to a fine point at the outer edge.

It would be almost criminal to overlook the victory roll hairstyle, which was a nod to the men fighting in the war. Ladies with mid-length to long hair 'rag rolled' their hair at a time when curlers and hairpins were in short supply. To give rag rolling a go:

- Cut an old tea towel into 2-inch (5 cm) thick strips
- Wash and towel dry your hair and add some mousse to the ends
- Take medium-sized sections of damp hair, wind them around a piece of rag (no higher than chin level) and tie the rag in a knot. Repeat this all the way around
- Use a hairdryer on a low setting to dry your hair
- Sleep in the rag rollers
- When you wake up, remove the rags and hey presto, lovely curly hair.
- Add a light spritz of hairspray if needed.

WELL-PADDED

Whatever you're wearing, ladies, don't forget to include shoulder pads for a sure-fire way to add a little forties style to your blouses, jackets or dresses. Gentlemen can complete their look with a natty tie pin and a good-sized wrist watch. Wide boys and spivs were known for their immaculate presentation, which included well-groomed, thin moustaches, and made it a requirement to doff their fedora to the ladies at every opportunity!

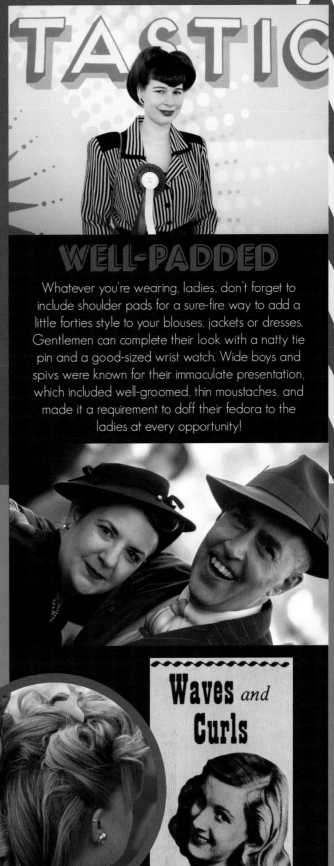

Waves and **Curls**

make your hair alluring . . .

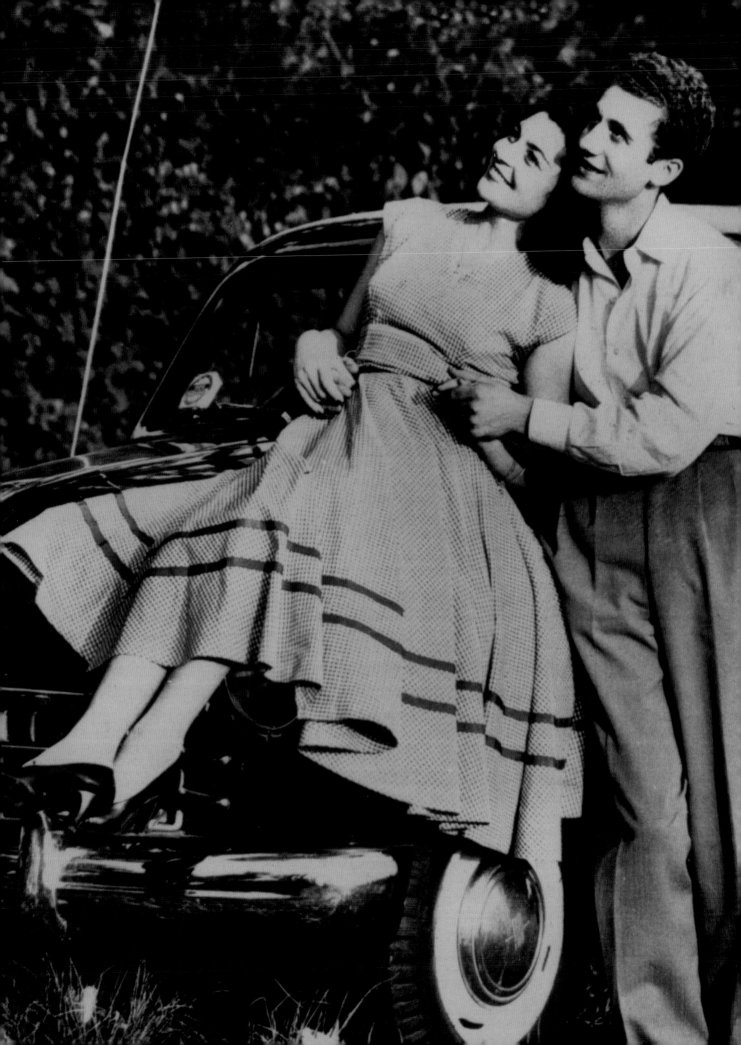

The 1950s

*T*he dawn of the new decade saw the shadows of the war fading and, with the opening the Festival of Britain in 1951, people's spirits were ignited by hope for a brighter and safer future. As fashion houses around the world reopened for business, designs were dominated by the great Parisian couturiers and the 'New Look', launched by Christian Dior in 1947, continued to be a huge influence until the mid-fifties.

After years of sensible dressing and minimal use of fabric, both women and men reached for luxury fabrics and favoured previously considered excesses, such as pockets and trims, but most of all colour. The fashion palette had been limited for some time and the fifties brought a wide variety of shades for clothes, including the ice-cream parlour pastels used for the emerging trend for separates as well as elegant evening wear. In addition, the decade saw the emergence of the working woman and also the birth of the 'teenager', with young people earning their own income and demanding their own identity and style. Men also became more fashion conscious, but the most significant development of the period was the arrival of the Teddy Boys. They were generally young men from working class backgrounds who adopted styles inspired by the dandies of the Edwardian period as part of their identity.

The 1950s had a diversity in fashion choice not seen for over a decade. Key pieces defined the fifties silhouette, such as the Capri pant that became the ultimate slim-line sexy trouser. Finishing anywhere from just below the knee to just above the ankle, the Capri pant was part of a collection by Sonja de Lennart. Her designs became a fashion must-have when Audrey Hepburn wore clothes styled from the Capri collection in the 1953 film, *Roman Holiday*.

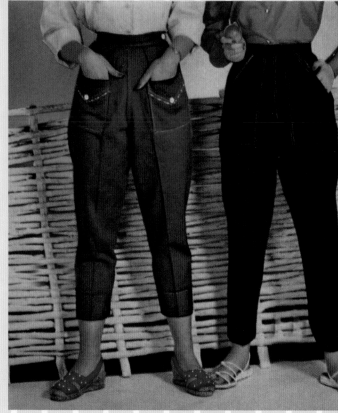

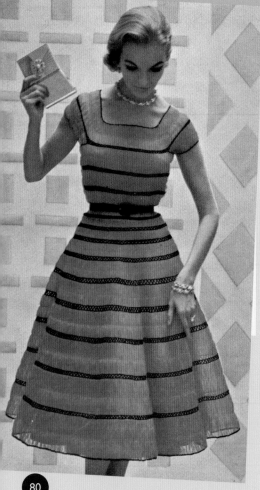

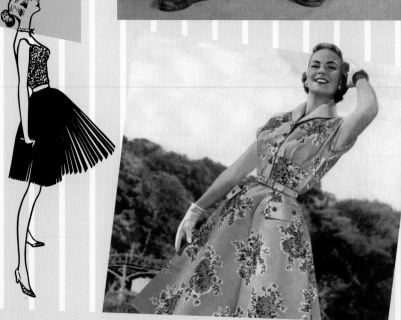

The next iconic fashion piece of the decade was the full skirt. Whether worn as a separate or as part of a dress, the skirt finished just below the knee with generous amounts of fabric that helped to create the shape. It was often worn with a netted underskirt and with the waist cinched in with a belt.

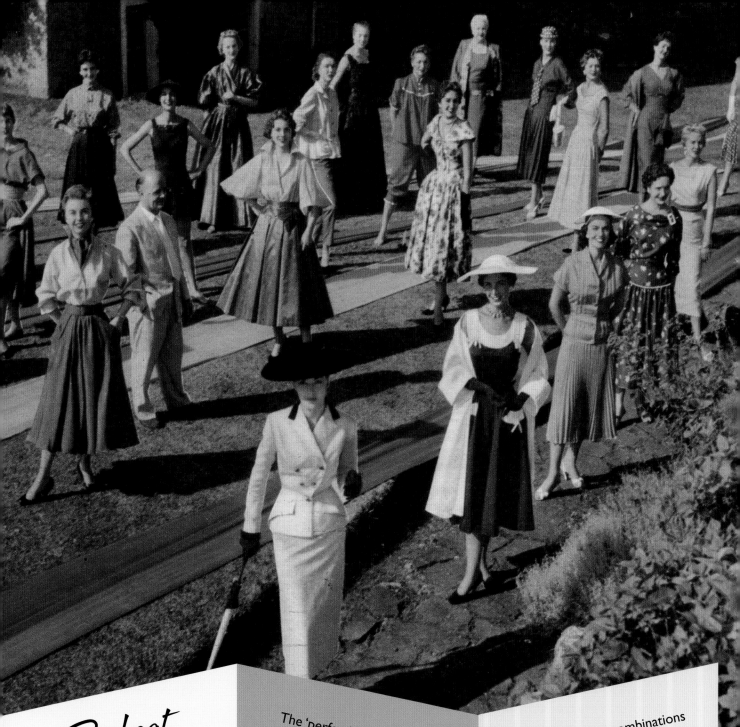

Perfect Housewives

A woman's wardrobe was in sharp focus in the fifties. Feminine elegance was the order, restoring the hourglass silhouette with the emphasis placed on delicate detailing, which could be added to cuffs, hems and décolletage.

The 'perfect' housewife was expected to look appealing at all times. 'House clothes' were ready-to-wear pieces that were less glamorous in both detail and fabric than special-occasion made-to-measure outfits. Typically a cotton or woolmix, a house dress would be sleeveless (or cap/three-quarter length) with a scoop or square neck, cinched at the waist with a pencil or A-line skirt shape.

Blouse and skirt combinations copied the house dress, although both might be button through. These were practical for doing light cleaning duties or cooking your husband's dinner (wearing an apron, of course) and still allowed you to look stylish. All aspects of home entertaining required a more formal style.

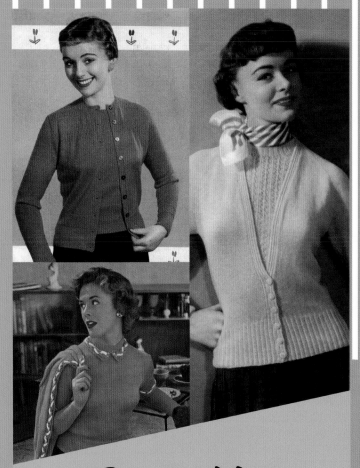

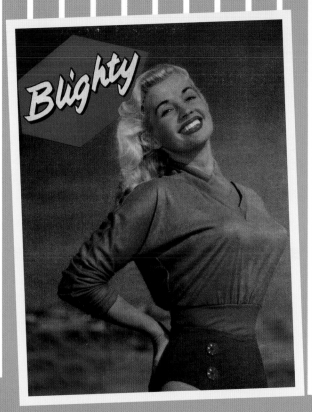

Set & Match

Nothing says fifties fashion like cardigans or twinsets. The term 'sweater girl' was first used in reference to Lana Turner in her tight-fitting knitted top in the film, *They Won't Forget*, in 1937, and the popularity of tight-fitting knitted tops showing off womanly curves went from strength to strength. During the 50s sexy knitwear was even more celebrated, being worn by screen goddesses such as Grace Kelly, Marilyn Monroe and Doris Day. The two-piece trend was huge and has stood the test of time to the present day.

Pastel or primary colours were most suited to the fashion feel of the fifties. The twinset typically consisted of a sleeveless crew-neck vest with matching cardigan, which was finished with delicate buttons or beading. Individual cardigans finished at the waist and had three-quarter or wrist-length sleeves. Knits tended to be fine rather than chunky and made from silks, rayon and jersey wool.

The fit of the twin set was vital to the look; it was intended to be figure hugging rather than hanging loose on the body. What was worn underneath was integral to creating the right shape. In 1953, underwear manufacturer Triumph launched its 'cone bra', which became affectionately known as the 'bullet bra'.

As the name suggests, the bra created a pointy, bullet shape and the cups were usually decorated with concentric circles or spirals to the nipple. The popularity of this bra design faded towards the end of the decade, but saw a resurgence in the eighties when Madonna wore a Jean Paul Gaultier version as outerwear.

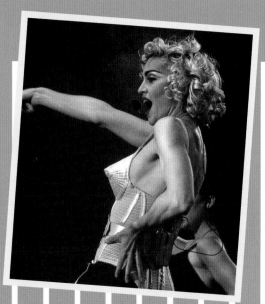

Coat Couture

A good coat that was warm, looked stylish and remained in fashion was important in the fifties. The swing coat, sometimes referred to as the 'trapeze', was an A-shape design often with a large collar, two large front-fastening buttons and three-quarter-length flared sleeves with a hemline finishing just below the knee. It was designed to complement the full skirts of the decade as well as being a practical wardrobe staple for fashion-conscious ladies who were contributing to the post-war 'baby boom'. These styles have remained popular, with original coats of quality being made from cashmere, wool and tweed. Wrap coats with wide tie belts came in a variety of materials and often had wide shawl collars.

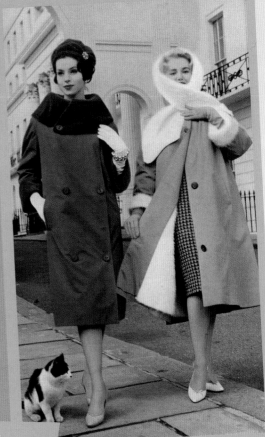

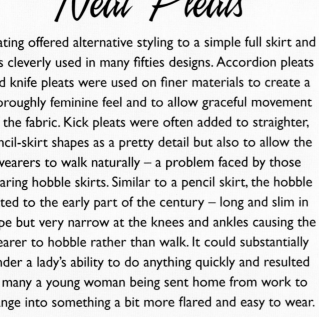

Get the Look with Hannah

Short cape-style coats flatter those wishing to accentuate their waist and are best worn with pencil skirts with a rear box pleat to balance the overall shape of your outfit.

Neat Pleats

Pleating offered alternative styling to a simple full skirt and was cleverly used in many fifties designs. Accordion pleats and knife pleats were used on finer materials to create a thoroughly feminine feel and to allow graceful movement of the fabric. Kick pleats were often added to straighter, pencil-skirt shapes as a pretty detail but also to allow the wearers to walk naturally – a problem faced by those wearing hobble skirts. Similar to a pencil skirt, the hobble dated to the early part of the century – long and slim in shape but very narrow at the knees and ankles causing the wearer to hobble rather than walk. It could substantially hinder a lady's ability to do anything quickly and resulted in many a young woman being sent home from work to change into something a bit more flared and easy to wear.

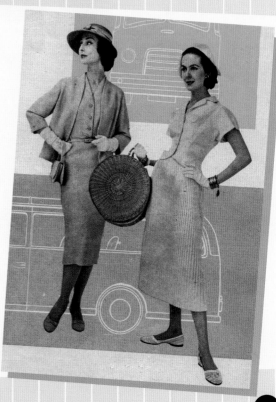

1950s Men's Day Wear

Whilst women were being physically constrained to attain an hour-glass shape, men's fashions were a lot more relaxed, with the term 'smart-casual' really coming into effect. Many men had spent years in uniform and longed for a time when comfort was a priority, and jackets and trousers did not need to match. The colour palette reflected this with unobtrusive 'earthy' colours, particularly brown. Grey also featured heavily in middle-class US corporate work wear.

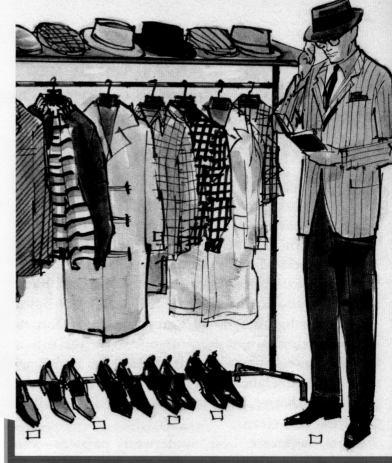

Suits US Style

America was forced to define its own fashion style in the 1950s, having been cut off from Europe during the war. Stateside came into its own at this time, leading the way with affordable off-the-peg casual wear. Double-breasted jackets became less popular with the two- or three- button single-breasted option being regarded as much more stylish. Shoulders remained broad but jacket length was reduced and collars made shorter and wider to expose more of the shirt underneath.

Pleated Trousers

Men's trousers became slightly fuller in the fifties with a more exaggerated turn-up depth and trouser length finishing on the shoe with no excess. This was in contrast to the mark of a bespoke trouser, which would typically finish on a slant. The UK turned trouser pleats (either one or two) inwards (forward) rather than outwards (reverse), as on the continent, and waistlines tended to sit in a natural position.

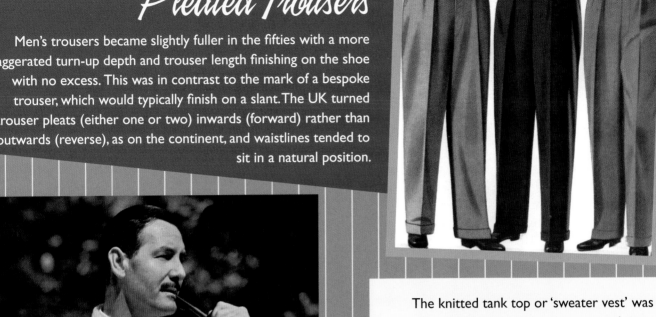

The knitted tank top or 'sweater vest' was favoured by many younger men and was largely worn with a shirt but no tie. The emergence of the American 'Ivy League' colleges in 1954 launched the 'preppy' look, which embraced sleeveless knitwear as part of the fashion subculture.

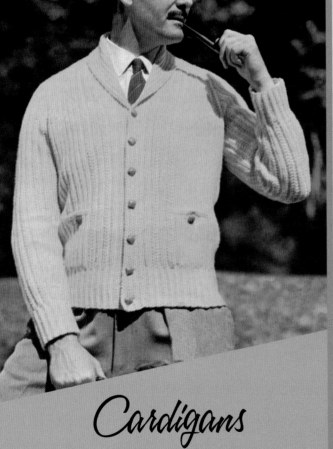

Cardigans

Cardigans became an acceptable alternative to the sports jacket and were similarly worn with a shirt and tie. Colour choices in knitwear for men were far more stimulating than those available in alternative day wear during the fifties and came in a variety of knitted styles. With women reinstated at home, knitting became a practical pastime and so to wear a piece of handmade stylish knitwear became an iconic symbol of domestic bliss.

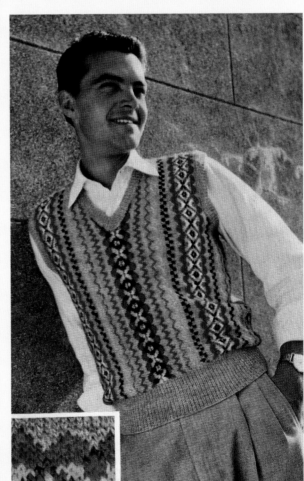

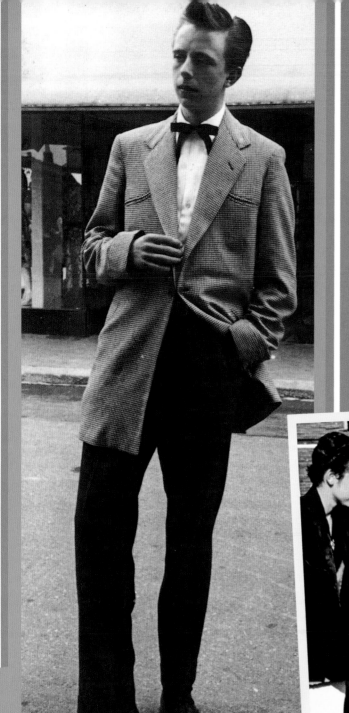

Return of the Beau

The 1950s saw the influential fashion magazine *Harper's Bazaar* announce that there was to be a 'return of the beau', which signified the creation of the 'New Edwardian Look' for men. This brought together the luxury and excess of Edwardian men's fashion with exaggerated shapes. Jackets became much longer and were edged in velvet around the collars and lapels as well as sporting velvet-covered French or ticket pockets and covered buttons. Trousers finished on the ankle exposing the socks, which were either dazzling white or a vibrant eye-catching colour to draw attention to chunky-soled lace-up shoes and slip-ons.

Teddy Boy

The Teddy Boy style was expensive, but with the youth of the day joining the workforce, the fashion was considered a means of breaking away from the past and creating a teenage identity. Slim-fitting, long-length drape jackets were worn with loose-fit white shirts, heavily embroidered waistcoats and drainpipe trousers, which often finished to expose the customary white socks.

In 1956, the film *Blackboard Jungle* premiered in South London. It detailed the plight of a dedicated teacher charged with bringing order to a class of unruly teenagers and ended to the song *Rock Around the Clock*, which saw the cinema audience of Teddy Boys and Girls dancing in the aisles. When cinema staff attempted to stop them, they rioted and ripped up the cinema seats with flick knives, earning the subculture a reputation that would precede them.

Easy Outer Wear

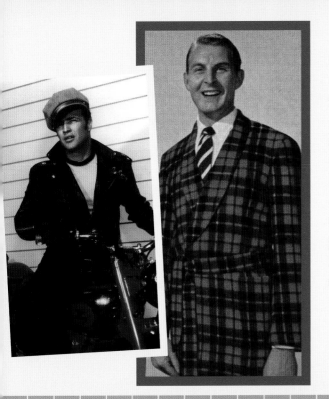

Shorter, casual jackets became a staple in the fashionable man's wardrobe with American checked hunting jackets and pea coats being most associated with the decade. Film rebels like James Dean and Marlon Brando (far left), were held responsible for the decline in leather jacket sales as conservative types feared their reputations might suffer if they adopted the denim jeans, white T-shirt and leather jacket bad-boy look. This soon changed as the look grew to be regarded as both sexy and iconic and is now considered a timeless style choice.

Perhaps without quite so much sex appeal, the duffle coat was still an integral part of fashion as surplus navy stock from World War II appeared in shops throughout the fifties. Its simplicity in design and the bonus of durability made it practical to wear. The duffle was made from a rough fabric called duffel from the town of Duffel in Belgium.

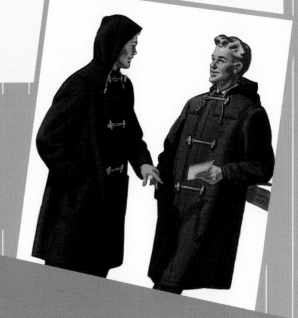

Banking on Style

Britain was on the verge of bankruptcy after the war and it wasn't until 1950 that the economy started to take a turn for the better. This led to the spread of the high-street bank, which in turn played a part in influencing fashion. Banking was an almost exclusively male environment which demanded attire that reflected the formality and sensible attitude required to work in the sector. The white-collar worker was just that, typically sporting a black single-breasted suit with high-waisted, slightly tapered trousers and a white-collar shirt. Ties were most often plain and the pervading headwear was the bowler. With the exception of the headwear, this look has remained synonomous with city workers around the world to the present day.

1950s *Women's Evening Wear*

Mid-century entertainment for many revolved around the cocktail party and was an ideal forum for social networking and to display a 'trophy wife'. This term is thought to have been first used in a 1950's article in *The Economist*. Women's fashion was dictated by men for most of the decade and this period encapsulates the idea of the 'ultimate housewife' whose sole purpose was to maintain high standards of appearance in her home, her children and herself. However, there is a saccharin charm about women's evening-wear design which embraces and celebrates the female form in all its glory.

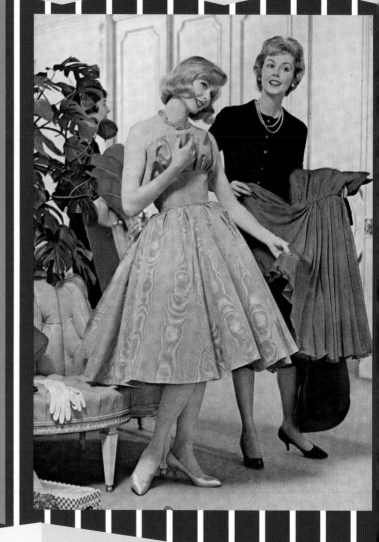

Shaken and Stirred

The cocktail dress was a shorter and less elaborate form of ball gown, which could be worn to attend a party in a less formal setting, such as in the home. If you couldn't quite afford couture, you would shop off-the-rail or show off your dressmaking skills or those of a local seamstress by creating your own from a pattern.

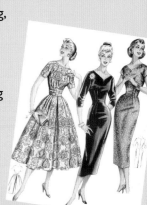

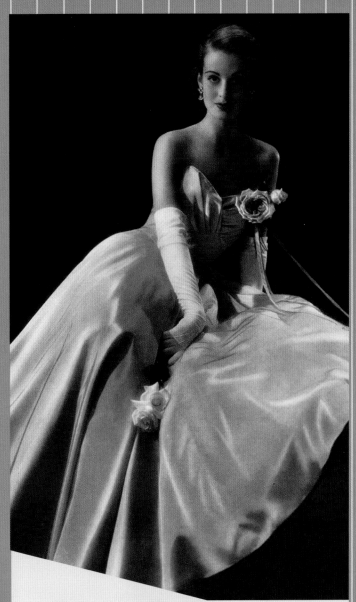

Much like the 1920s, evening wear was heavily embellished with sequins and beads. The removable waist corsage was also commonplace as was the use of fast evolving man-made fabrics. Nylon, which had been used for parachutes during the war, was continually refined and used extensively in the 1950s. Most notably, nylon was the material used to hold together the corset structure of the strapless dress.

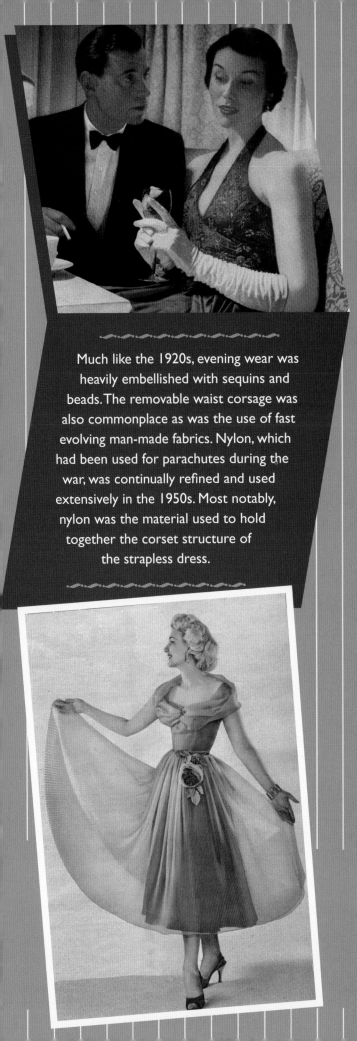

Glam Gals!

For many women the 1950s reinforced the importance of always making an effort with your appearance, no matter what your age. Designers such as Cristóbal Balenciaga, Hubert De Givenchy, Pierre Balmain and Yves Saint Laurent were all entering the fashion arena in the 1950s. In addition, high-street labels like Harrods and Harvey Nichols and Californian company Lilli Ann had the most sought-after designers for high-quality women's wear.

Grace of Lace

Lace is a material which looks chic and elegant on women of all age groups. Lace production has firm roots in Europe: prior to the 1950s, there was a thriving market for handmade and machine lace production in the town of Honiton, Devon and the city of Nottingham in the UK. Yet the decade saw the demise of UK-manufactured lace, with much of the production being carried out abroad. The delicate nature of lace meant dresses and skirts made from the material were often designed over block colour slip dresses or shapes to preserve modesty, or created in multiple layers to add volume.

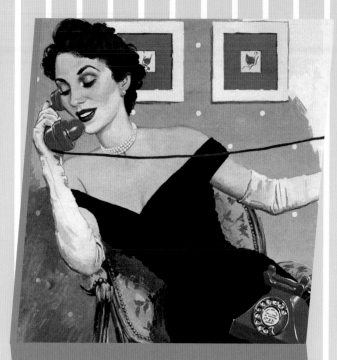

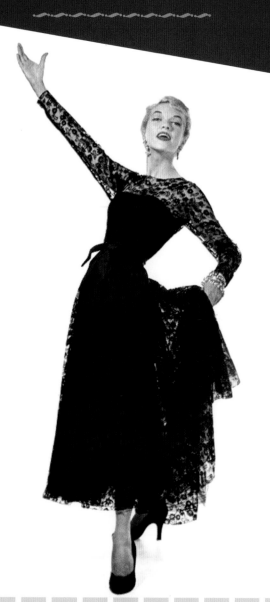

Get the Look with Hannah

During this decade evening wear was all about variations in the neckline, and it is helpful to consider your face and body shape before deciding what style might flatter you most. A smaller frame and bust can carry a strapless or off-the-shoulder look more elegantly than those who require more support to lift the bust and define the waist. Those falling into the latter category should avoid the boat-cut neckline and opt for a sleeveless but wide-strap deeper V-neck to elongate the neck and accentuate the décolletage. Halter-neck dresses can be flattering on both smaller and larger frames but require an upright posture to create the most flattering silhouette.

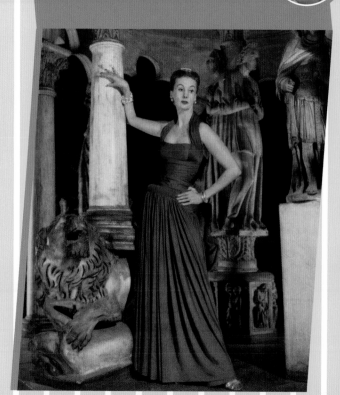

Fabulously Faux

Real fur was expensive, difficult to store and becoming controversial in the 1950s, and so with advances in man-made materials, faux fur found its place in the fashion world. Leopard print was a firm favourite as an evening coat, signifying the exotic with a bold pattern. This print sat well against primary colours such as red and green, which were popular for evening dresses, alongside the obligatory black. As wearing gloves was still mandatory fashion etiquette in the 1950s, sleeve lengths on coats most often stopped short of the wrist.

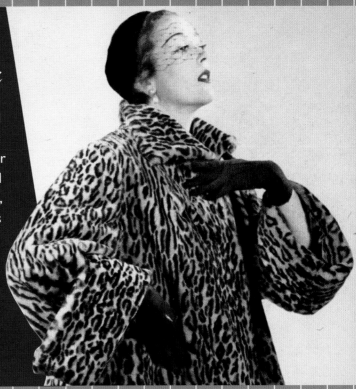

Shape Shifters

Evening-wear shapes ranged from the iconic Dior 'New Look', which consisted of a cinched waist and wide flared skirt, right through to the sheath, which might fantail at the calf, and so evening gowns often required excessive layers of petticoats to provide lift and movement. It was essential that the underskirts kept their shape so sugar solution or starch would be used to stiffen them.

Belle of the Ball

Adults wanted to maintain the rules of 'proper' social etiquette in the 1950s and whilst rock 'n' roll and youth movements dominated the media, the sophistication of grown-up evening wear lent itself to the ballroom – this, after all, was where the ball gown was designed to be seen. Although variations of ball gowns had been worn since the early 1800s as evening wear, the exaggerated wide skirt shape complemented the trends of the era perfectly and was most often designed as a floor-length gown.

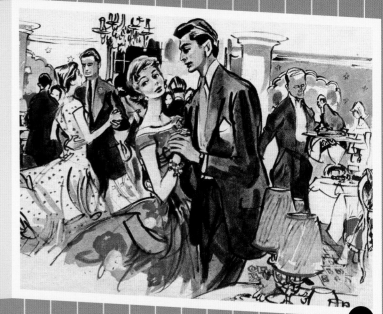

1950s Men's Evening Wear

Much like today, a good wardrobe had staple pieces for both day and evening wear. These offered mix and match options in keeping with the new 'ready-to-wear' shopping experience but without totally relinquishing all elements of convention. It was important to own suits for different occasions: for business and semi-formal wear, and a tuxedo for black-tie engagements.

Top Coats

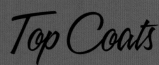

Overcoats fell into categories with the Paletot coat being paired with black tie for evening wear (offered as a single- or double-breasted coat with a hint of a waistline) or the more casual double-breasted Ulster overcoat. Both coats were tailored with enough fabric to allow for ease of movement over a suit. They were generally made from heavy materials, such as tweed or wool, so were uncomfortable in warm weather, creating the need for lightweight versions like the Ulsterette.

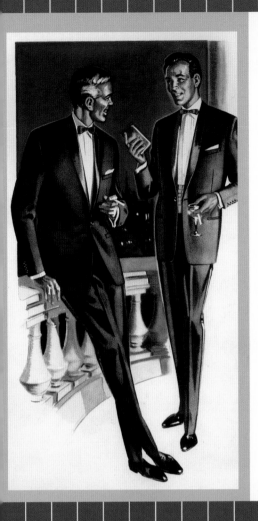

The Tuxedo

Although men's fashion had evolved over time, the tuxedo remained an important part of evening-wear code and a symbol of fashion formality. However, the cut had become svelter by the early 1950s, losing the wide lapels and broad shoulders in favour of narrower and sharper edges with a shawl collar. During the latter part of the decade, evening wear began to borrow a little more from the Edwardian beau influence and paralleled the increasingly ornate jackets and waistcoats being seen on Teddy Boys. The satin cummerbund was reinstated and sat atop shirts with lace embroidery and soft ruffles, creating a much softer edge to men's tailoring and giving the overall look a more delicate finish.

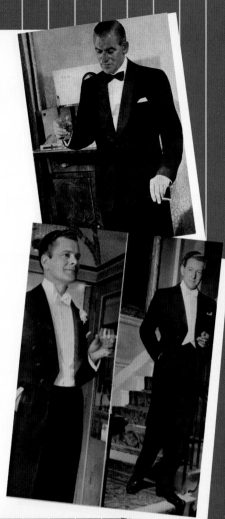

And the award goes to ...

If female film stars were watched for their style choices in the 1950s, the same could be said of the men. Frank Sinatra, Dean Martin, Sammy Davis Jr and Peter Lawford were always immaculately dressed in sharp suits and were amongst some of the biggest names of the time. Endlessly snapped in the company of the rich and famous (if not sometimes dangerous) their attire was constantly scrutinized and what they were wearing had a strong influence on the fast-evolving ready-to-wear designs being manufactured. Revered as playboys of the day, when the magazine named *Playboy* created its iconic logo in 1953 it chose a rabbit to represent friskiness and a formal bow tie to signify masculine elegance and sophistication. By 1959, the more elaborate detailing of evening wear was spotted on fashion-conscious celebrities at the Academy Awards Oscars ceremony, and, like today, had an immediate impact on consumer demand for clothes.

Italy provided the catalyst for further changes and alternatives in men's wear design at the end of the decade. Italian designers created suits in lighter fabrics with shorter, more fitted jackets and narrow lapels, which could be worn as day wear as well as for formal occasions. This set the precedent for the change in fashion attitudes that would take over in the next decade.

1950s Shoes

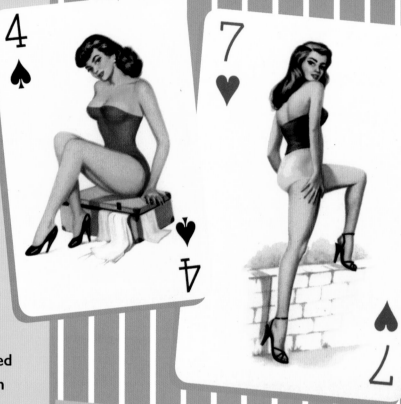

In 1953 Roger Vivier developed a close working relationship with Christian Dior to breathe new life into an old shoe design – the stiletto. The pencil-thin, towering heel of the stiletto remains a shoe closely associated with a woman's sexual image. Although women had been known to wear a version of a stiletto as far back as Victorian times, the technology to produce a stable, thin, high heel was not mastered until the 1950s. Lessons were offered to help ladies walk properly in them and there were always complaints about the damage that the sharp heels of stilettos did to flooring.

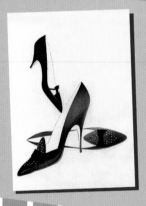

Mehmet Kurdash founded Gina Shoes in 1954, naming the company as a tribute to his favourite actress, Gina Lollobrigida. The shoes were worn by celebrities and royalty for decades and the company still operates from its original factory in Dalston, East London.

Pump it up

In stark contrast to the towering heel, the ballet pump was a firm favourite throughout the 1950s. The slip-on pump worked well with Capri pants as well as dresses, and appealed to both the younger and the older consumer.

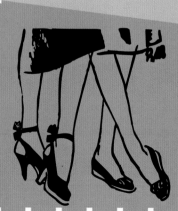

The traditional design for men's lace-up brogues remained very popular throughout the 1950s. Companies such as Tricker's embraced the trend for smart casual shoes.

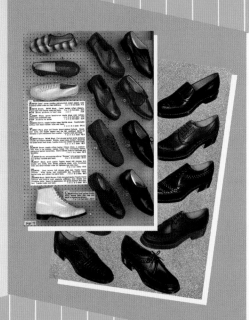

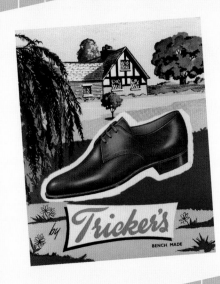

Jeepers Creepers

Both formal and casual footwear for men was influenced by styles seen in Europe, with many British manufacturers creating slip-on designs. This was a welcome change from the all-encompassing lace-up boot worn extensively in the previous decade. However, the biker boot was still worn by male Rockers.

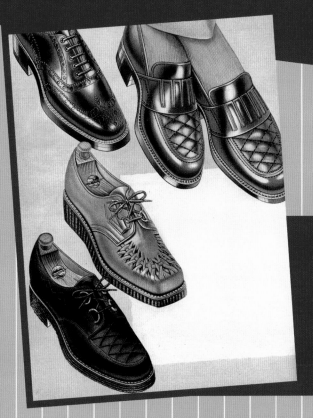

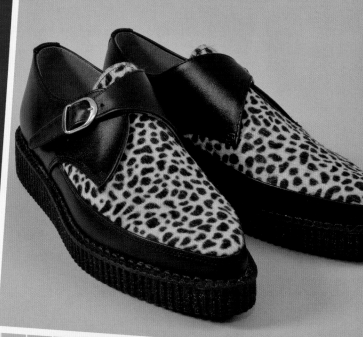

Creepers (above) earned their name due to the silent footsteps made by the wearers of these crepe-soled shoes. The thick platform sole also offered the Teddy Boys and Rockers a few extra inches in height. Creepers were sold in a whole host of colours. In 1956, Elvis famously sang about his *Blue Suede Shoes*, which saw a surge in sales of creepers in this colour and material.

Leisure wear combined functionality with good design and became hugely popular in the 1950s. With growing demands from the teenage consumer, the USA was the first to seize the chance to create fashion specifically for this new group. Sport and leisure wear gave teenagers the opportunity to turn their backs on old-fashioned formal and casual wear labels and to identify themselves as sassy and vibrant by wearing more modern and youthful designs.

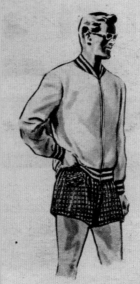

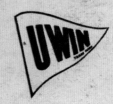

Make Leisure a Pleasure in UWIN

Model A.2017
This attractive casual jacket of knitted fleecy-backed cotton, White trimmed contrast, can also be obtained in Scarlet, Royal or Saxe trimmed contrast. From 35s. 0d. each

Model C.8781
Beach shorts in Tartan shades are of rayon cotton. From 25s. 0d. pair

In case of difficulty write to:
PUBLICITY MANAGER, UWIN HOUSE,
35 ST. PAUL'S CHURCHYARD · LONDON · E.C.4

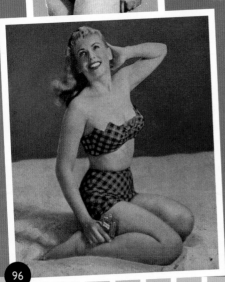

Bikini Battle

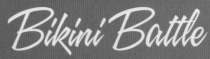

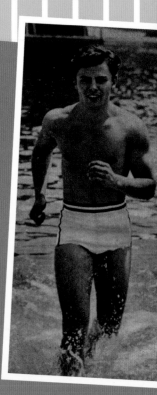

Although the female form was accentuated in most clothing design, opinions differed as to what was appropriate when it came to swim wear. Going to the seaside was a big part of 1950s life and swim wear continued to raise eyebrows. During the early part of the decade, the one-piece design was favoured; it tended to be cut low to the thigh and have a relatively high front and back. Navy blue was a popular colour choice, with floral or nautical patterns or detailing. The middle to the end of the decade saw the bikini become popular, although the waist was usually high, a look closely associated with pin-up girls. With more families able to take holidays, men began wearing swimming trunks in a short style, which sparked many debates on male modesty.

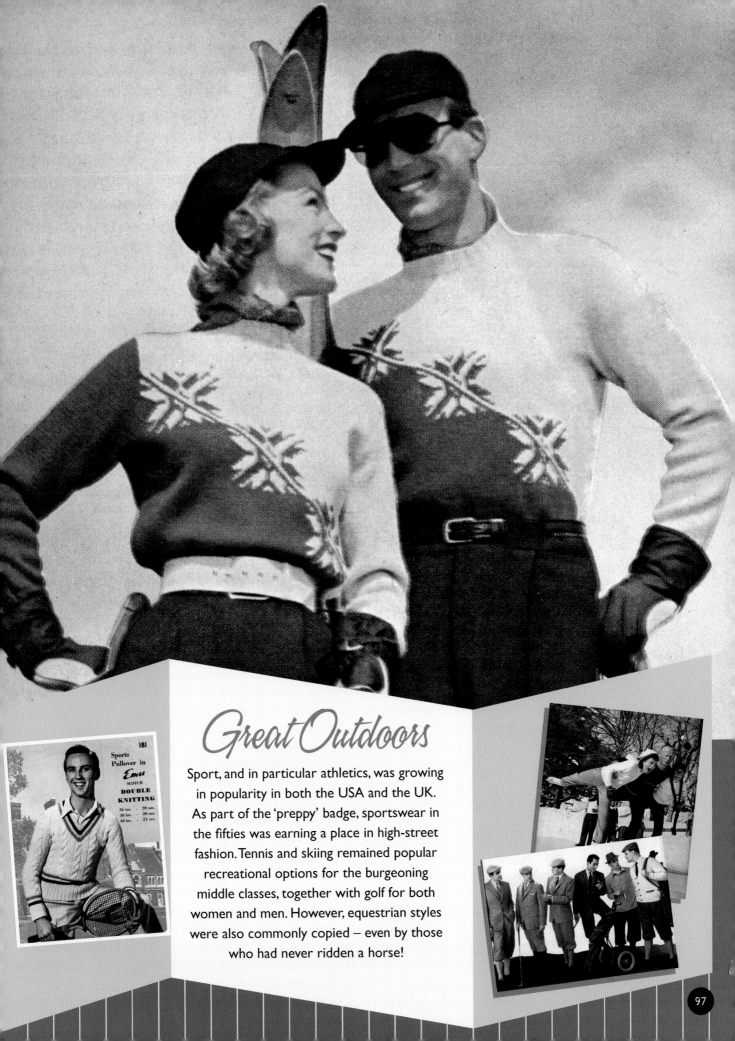

Great Outdoors

Sport, and in particular athletics, was growing in popularity in both the USA and the UK. As part of the 'preppy' badge, sportswear in the fifties was earning a place in high-street fashion. Tennis and skiing remained popular recreational options for the burgeoning middle classes, together with golf for both women and men. However, equestrian styles were also commonly copied – even by those who had never ridden a horse!

181
Sports
Pullover in
Emu
SCOTCH
**DOUBLE
KNITTING**
36 ins. · 20 ozs.
38 ins. · 20 ozs.
40 ins. · 21 ozs.

1950s *Accessories*

To complete any authentic fifties outfit a hat was essential. Ladies wore tri-corner ensembles with pretty embellishments, Juliet caps and berets. There was also a surge in designs featuring flamboyant marabou and ostrich feathers with some hats literally covered in them. Knitted hats were a more affordable option, although they were considerably less glamorous – more functional than fashionable. Head scarves in the fifties provided women of all ages with a simple alternative to wearing a hat and proved to be both a style statement and a great way to protect hairstyles from the elements.

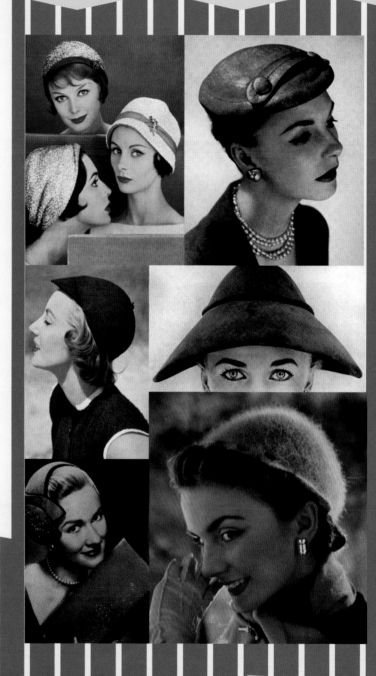

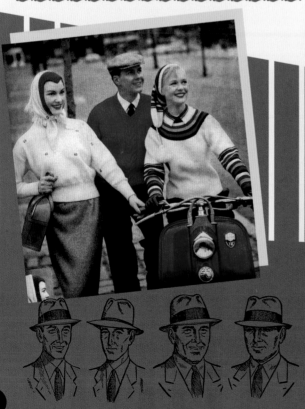

For men, the wide-brimmed fedora and the trilby continued to be fashionable, whilst the bowler was the headwear of choice for formal occasions and was associated with the typical British gent.

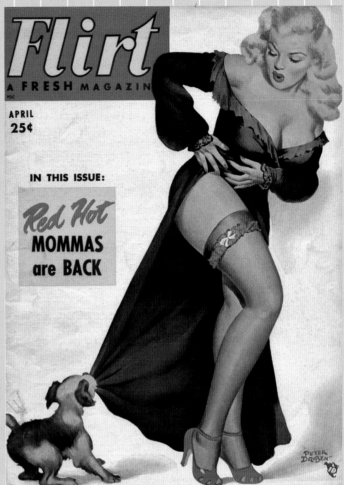

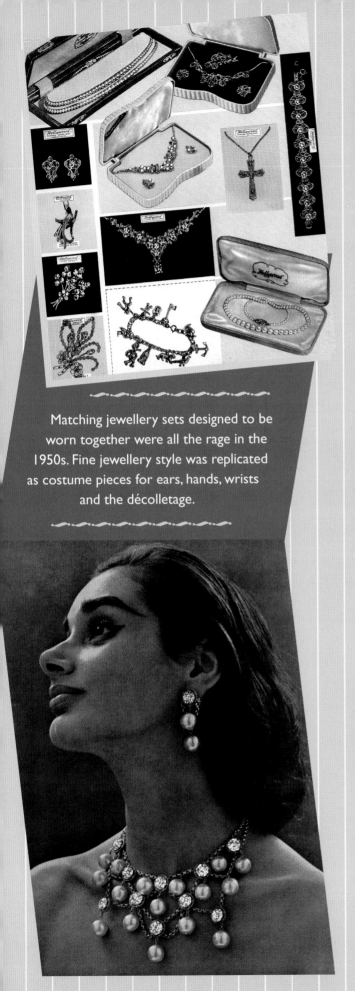

Matching jewellery sets designed to be worn together were all the rage in the 1950s. Fine jewellery style was replicated as costume pieces for ears, hands, wrists and the décolletage.

Morley ran its campaigns for stockings using pin-up images, becoming one of the best-selling manufacturers of the time. Rival DuPont focused on the durability of nylon and chose a scientific approach to its advertising.

Men's Underwear

It was common for men to wear both vests and long johns (a type of thermal legging) at the start of the decade – a habit from the war years. However, as fashion changed, this was considered prudish. Underwear using Aertex allowed men to remain fresher in their clothes, and gradually vests and long undershorts were ditched in favour of Y-fronts. By 1959, helped by the continental influence, briefs and boxer shorts were standard wear.

1950s Get the Look with Hannah

Mention fifties make-up to anyone with only the vaguest knowledge of the period and you can bet they will mention eyeliner. Well-groomed eyebrows, neutral, muted eyeshadow tones, minimal blusher, pastel or red shades on the lips and eyeliner really make the look.

Cat-eye glasses shout 1950s and are a sure-fire way to make a statement with your look, whatever the weather.

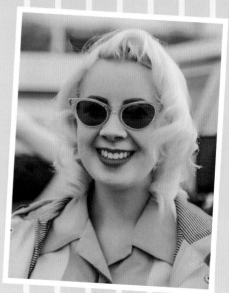

JOHN ANTHONY

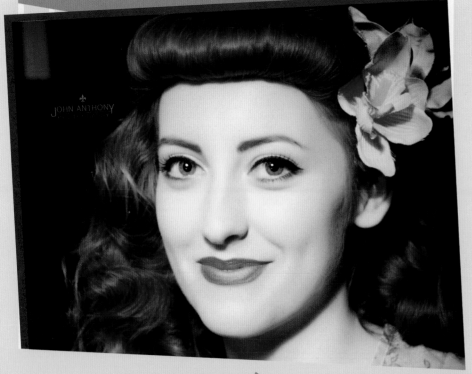

Heels and Hose

The Cuban heel stocking looks stunning teamed with skyscraper heels. Original stock is relatively easy to find and often comes in attractive packaging. As the design has remained timeless, you should be able to pick up modern-day variations as well as pantyhose if you require something a little more snug from your hosiery.

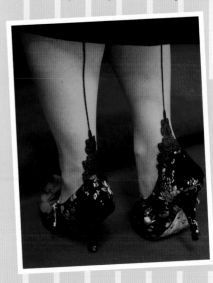

Eye Lines

Applying eyeliner can take some time to master. Use a fine-tipped brush with a gel-based liner. Follow the natural contour of the bottom of the outer corner of the eye with your liner. Next, draw a thin line along the upper lash line to meet the bottom line to make an inverted V. Fill in the V to create a fabulous fifties flick.

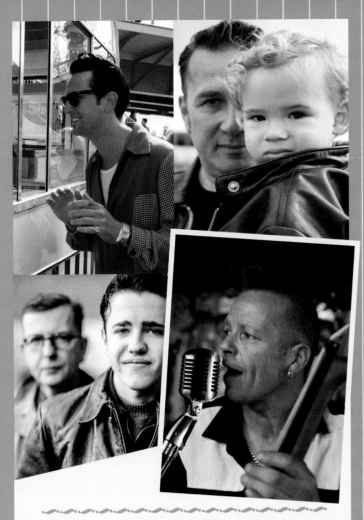

His Hair

In the fifties men wore a wider variety of hairstyles than ever before. With music and fashion dictating which 'group' they were part of, their hair would be styled accordingly. Elvis sported the Pompadour, which saw the hair over the forehead swept up into a quiff, the sides combed backwards and all held in place with a hair product, such as Brylcreem, and the back combed neatly downwards.

The DA (duck's ass), although first sported in the 1940s, was closely associated with the Teddy Boys and Rockers and named for its resemblance to the aquatic bird's derriere. Similar to the Pompadour, the top was piled high and the sides greased back. However, a distinct seam was created at the rear, which gave the style its name. Those not affiliated to these two groups may have sported a crew cut or flat top but, regardless of their 'gang', men's hair was slicked into shape.

Her Hair

Ladies' hairstyles demanded length with the chignon and the front quiff ponytail representing sophistication and playfulness respectively. For the latter, take a small square portion of hair from the front middle section of your hairline. Holding the hair upwards, gently backcomb the roots to give density and carefully smooth out any wispy hair with a bristle brush. Squirt with hairspray and curl the hair towards the back of your head into a small roll. Push the hair forwards a little to create a quiff shape and secure with hair pins on the inside of the roll. Take the remaining hair and pull back into a high ponytail. Secure with a hairband. Create a neat finish using hairspray to smooth back any flyaway hairs. For an additional twist, take a small section of the ponytail and wrap it around the hairband.

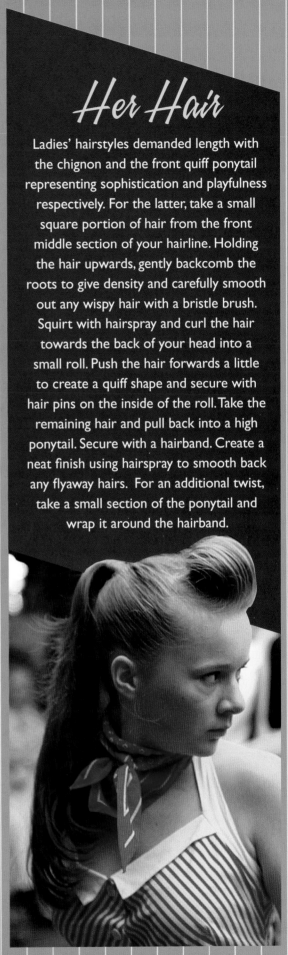

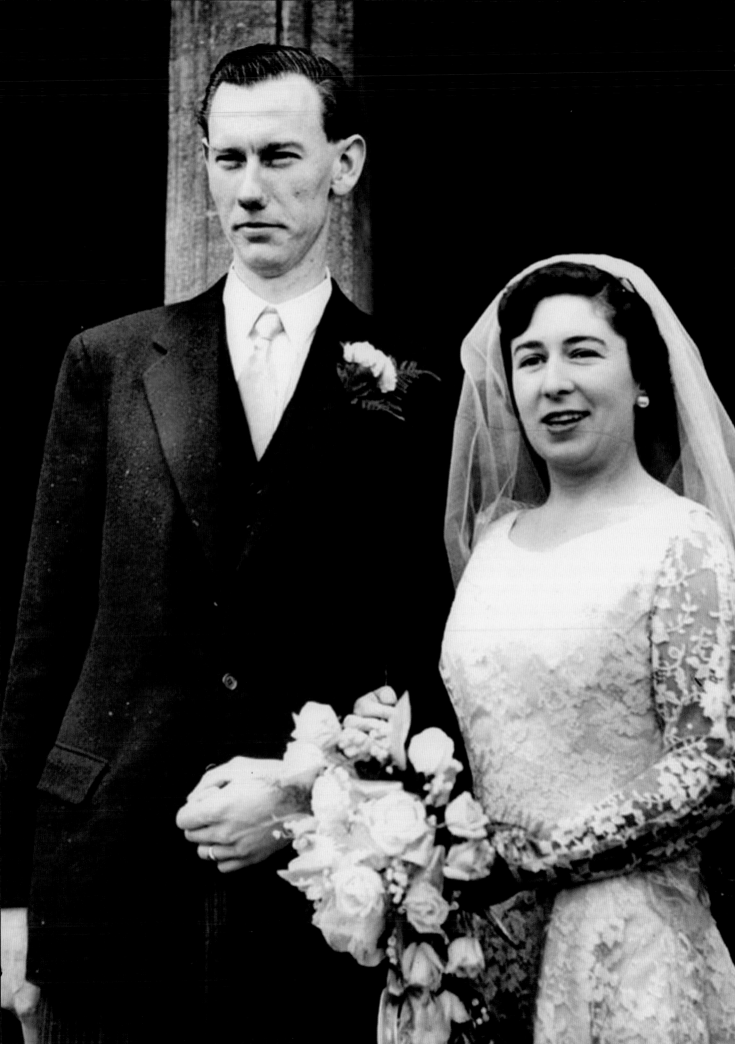

VINTAGE WEDDINGS

Get the Look with Hannah

The commercialization of weddings was first seized upon at the end of World War I in 1918 when the devastating loss of male lives made the prospect of finding a husband a challenge and the opportunity to be the ultimate vision of loveliness in a bridal gown imperative. Magazine articles were devoted to advice on how to find 'Mr Right' and what to do when the hunt was over, the quest to look your best at all times both before and, indeed, after your nuptials, and how to ensure you didn't lose your man to a more meticulously groomed rival. The sources of advice were endless, and by 1934 a publication called *Brides* was launched and went on to be credited for starting the proliferation of ubiquitous bridal shops that can be found around the world today.

With all eyes focused on the happy couple throughout their special day, not to mention the photographic reminders and the fact that the dress will probably be one of the most expensive fashion purchases the woman will ever make, getting the look right is always crucial! The key thing to bear in mind with any aspect of wedding fashion is not to get caught up in what might be 'in' right now and instead focus on what is best suited to you. As a make-up artist and stylist with years of experience working with brides, my advice is to always give detailed consideration to your height, body frame, hair length, face shape and skin tones as much as the time of year, time of day and location. Wearing 1950s stiletto heels when you are taller than the groom could be as much of a bad idea as choosing a spaghetti-strap flapper dress to wear in the snow!

Although the subject is far from exhaustive, the following pages provide a basic guide to the key elements of wedding fashion throughout the decades and aim to give you an idea of which era might work best for you.

1920s WEDDING

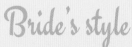

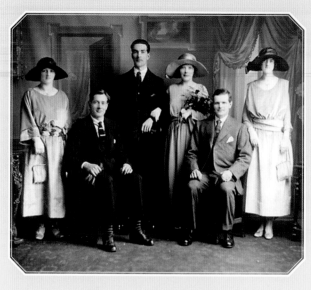

Bride's style

Styles from this period generally suit slender body shapes and smaller busts best. Modern backless, strapless bras or multiway bras are great for spaghetti strap or low back dresses. Materials like silk were popular embellished with lace, pearls, sequins and mother of pearl. Hem lengths varied, typically falling to mid-calf, but traditional shoes had a relatively low heel, so bear this in mind if you have a short stature as this may not be flattering. Mary Jane shoes offset a period style dress perfectly. Complementary lingerie would be silk camisoles and French knickers but to flatten your chest consider a bandeau bra.

Groom's style

Early 1920s style favours jackets and tails that button high on the chest with trousers that sit above the waistline, which are better suited to slender men. Styles from the late twenties have longer length jackets and Oxford bag trousers with turn ups, which can be flattering for men of a large stature. Heavy wool is the authentic material for the twenties accompanied by a shirt that is crisp, wingtip collar, bib front and cufflink fastened (preferably with monogrammed cufflinks). Socks were sometimes partially on show so consider sock suspenders to keep them high on the calf. Shoe styles will vary depending on the level of formality you are going for but Oxfords are the classic style.

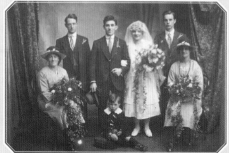

20s Checklist: Bride

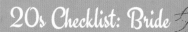

Dress material & shape: silk, satin; tubular; spaghetti strap
Dress colour: white
Dress neck: wide, round or square
Hem length: mid-calf to ankle
Headdress: cloche or Juliet cap
Shoes: Mary Jane style

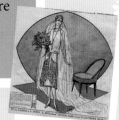

20s Checklist: Groom

Suit: single breasted; morning tailcoat; high waist trousers; military style; wide-notch lapels
Shirt: white cotton or silk with bib front and detachable wingtip collar
Neckwear: silk tie or cravat
Hat: top hat
Shoes: Oxfords; toe cap; two tone

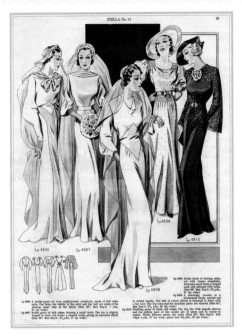

1930s WEDDING

Bride's style

Crinoline was a popular material for gowns in the early part of the decade but was soon overtaken by the demand for floor-length silk, satin and crepe dresses with long sleeves cut on the bias. The figure-hugging nature of this style means that getting your underwear correct is imperative. Authentic period lingerie consists of a brief bra and girdle and may well have included suspenders. Try to avoid foundation garments that are heavily embellished or trimmed with lace as this will show through delicate fabrics. Bridal shoes from the period are very decorative although bear in mind they will be largely covered by the dress.

30s Checklist: Bride

Dress material & shape: crinoline; bias cut; bell sleeves
Dress colour: white
Dress neck: high scoop; bateau
Hem length: ankle; floor
Headdress: tiaras; pill-box hat
Shoes: satin; round toe; embellishments

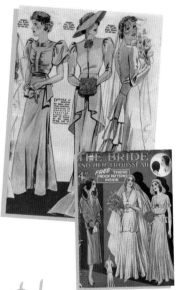

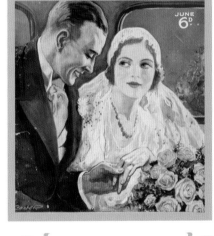

Groom's style

Very slender men can get 'lost' in decade-specific formal wear, which can be wide on the shoulders and have excess material so ensure that the suit fits well all over. Nipped-in waist jackets and tapered trousers were fashionable around the middle of the decade although waistlines still sat high on the body, which means this style will naturally lend itself best to gentlemen without protruding stomachs. Button-down, classic-cut shirts are easy to wear and work for both smaller and larger men. Cuffs should ideally be link fastened. Sock suspenders are good for keeping silk socks from sliding down whilst classic styles of shoes from the previous decades with soft, round toes will finish off the outfit perfectly. Match your hat to your outfit style and the season.

30s Checklist: Groom

Suit: single breasted; drape cut; shoulder pads; nipped-in waist jacket; tapered trousers
Shirt: classic fit; front button-down
Neckwear: geometric; bold-print ties
Hat: top hat; straw; fedora
Shoes: Oxfords; toe cap; two tone

1940s WEDDING

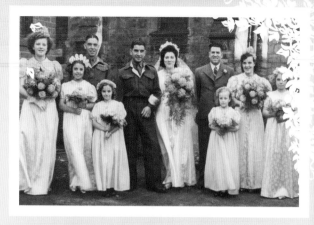

Bride's style

In a time so fraught with austerity and patriotism, the 1940s bride often chose simplicity in her wedding attire and elected to marry in a smart two-piece skirt suit instead of a traditional gown. In the absence of a bouquet try making a corsage, which can be worn on the lapel of your jacket and potentially replicated with a manly touch for the groom's buttonhole. Wedding dresses from this period are not overly detailed and will often be cut to flatter curves with no excess of material. This makes 1940s styles appealing to a wider audience than the previous two decades. Accentuating your figure will require a well-fitted bra, and a girdle with built-in suspenders will not only help flatten the stomach but allow you to wear nude plain-top stockings for an authentic finish. Round-toe court shoes are a simple, classic finish but you could add a touch of sparkle, with decorative shoe clips.

Groom's style

Men often married in their armed forces uniform but regular men's suits were cut in a more classic style during the forties, which generally means a loose-fit style. 'Demob' suits were issued to soldiers returning to Civvy Street but these were more often than not ill fitting and oversized for the lean frames of soldiers returning from the harshness of war, so bear this in mind if you have a compact or trim figure. A single-breasted jacket will flatter both small and large frames whilst the double-breasted jacket will give a more boxy finish to the upper body. However this style can make the midriff look larger which may not be welcome. As with most things 1940s, there isn't much in the way of detail so think creatively and add a point of interest with a patterned tie or breast-pocket handkerchief. Shoes were utilitarian so stick to classic lace-up styles with soft, round toes.

40s Checklist: Groom

Suit: single- or double-breasted; armed forces uniform
Shirt: armed forces shirt; classic-cut front button-down
Neckwear: plain or patterned
Hat: armed forces headwear; fedora
Shoes: military boots; round toe; two-eyelet lace ups

40s Checklist: Bride

Dress material & shape: parachute silk; two-piece skirt suit
Dress colour: white; cream; ivory
Dress neck: high scoop
Hem length: mid-calf to ankle
Headdress: tiara; flower band
Shoes: court shoe

1950s WEDDING

Bride's style

Wedding dresses got shorter in the 1950s, with popular hemlines finishing just below the knee. There was a fashion for sheer fabrics and lace, which will allow you to reveal more flesh whilst still retaining your modesty, and the favoured sweetheart neckline helps show off the dècolletage and elongate the neck, creating the illusion of height. Sleeveless dresses were not common but if you want to expose your arms choose a lace or sheer bolero that can be worn in a formal/religious setting and then taken off later in the day. High necklines will suit a smaller bust whilst more open necklines will flatter a larger chest. Whatever dress you choose, be sure to accentuate a small waist. Corsets can help you achieve this and can be worn independently or as part of the dress structure. With hem lengths shortened during this period, shoes were a prominent part of the bridal attire – look for kitten or mid-height stiletto heels with open or pointed toes to keep in style with the period.

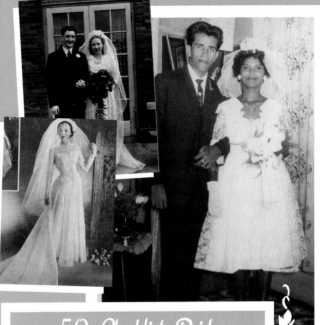

50s Checklist: Bride

Dress material & shape: lace; bell shape
Dress colour: white
Dress neck: sweetheart; bateau
Hem length: mid-calf to ankle
Headdress: bonnets; pill-box hat; tiara
Shoes: satin; pointed toe; kitten or stiletto heel

50s Checklist: Groom

Suit: single- or double-breasted; wide leg trousers
Shirt: classic front button-down
Neckwear: tie
Hat: none
Shoes: slip-ons; Oxfords

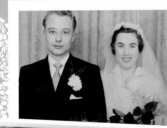

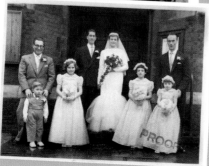

Groom's style

Menswear rules relaxed in the fifties and so a formal suit and tie are as accetable as a wedding ensemble as are tails. The boxy shape of a double- breasted suit will serve to emphasize a gent's physique whilst the slim-fitting single-breasted options can work for both small and large frames, so choose according to stature. Trousers should be wide in the leg with trouser cuffs resting on the shoes, which should be Oxfords. Those seeking a more striking look could consider a Teddy-boy suit with Edwardian influences, sporting a broad-cut drape jacket with velvet trim and drainpipe trousers complete, with exposed socks and creepers.

1960s WEDDING
Bride's style

1960s wedding dresses are simple in design with varying hem lengths. Brides with long, slim legs can get away with a sleeveless mini shift dress whilst those looking for more coverage can elect for a scoop-neck empire-line dress that finishes at the ankle. Foundation garments are structured and can be worn to control problem areas. Brassieres should lift the bust (in keeping with the period), and use shape-control knickers to instantly flatten and smooth the stomach and hips. Shoes evolved from pointed-toe kitten heels to a narrow heel with a small, square toe and then wide block heeled sling-backs with broad, round toes.

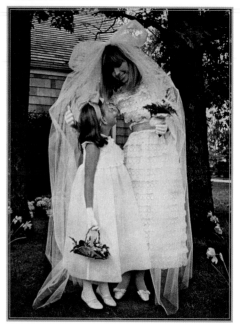

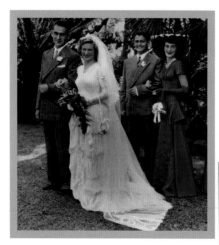

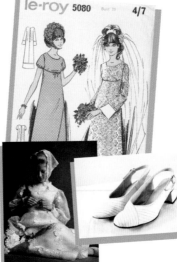

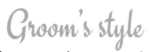

60s Checklist: Bride

Dress material & shape: synthetic materials, lace or satin; shift shape; empire line
Dress colour: white
Dress neck: mandarin collar; polo neck; high scoop
Hem length: from mini to ankle length
Headdress: bonnet
Shoes: round toe; sling-back

60s Checklist: Groom

Suit: slim fit; top hat; tails; flared trousers
Shirt: wide collars
Neckwear: cravat; slim ties
Hat: top hat
Shoes: Chelsea boots; slip-ons; pointed toe; Oxfords

Groom's style

Top hat and tails for the man on the street made a brief comeback to fashionable groom's wear in the sixties; however it was the Continent that provided the main influence for grooms and general menswear, with Italian slim-fit suits the order of the day. Bespoke tailoring will always provide the most complimentary fit for a man's suit so if your budget permits, go for something which will remain a classic and can be worn after the big day. Shoes should not be chunky, which is somewhat of a contrast to women's shoe shapes of the decade. Go for leather slip-ons or two-hole lace-up shoes, or Chelsea boots with a rounded point and low heel. Accessorize with a narrow silk tie.

1970s WEDDING

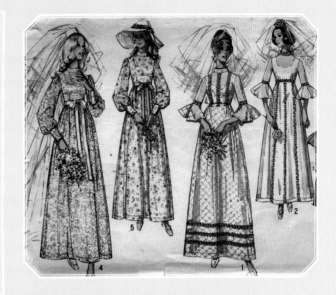

Bride's style

The seventies bridal look was inspired by Edwardian design and peppered with nostalgia and romance but the floor-sweeping gowns were given a period twist with stacked platform shoes. The kaftan-style dresses mean that women of all shapes and sizes can wear bridal outfits from this period but large ladies should bear in mind that free-shaped dresses can serve to increase the illusion of size. Foundation wear from the period has a strong emphasis on lace and so makes for pretty bridal lingerie. To contour your waist consider a basque with built-in suspenders, or a suspender belt teamed with classic briefs. Brides with a slender physique could consider a teddy to emulate the look of a camisole and French knickers. Seventies dresses rarely exposed the arms and were usually ankle length, which is great for those looking for modest attire or getting married in cool climates.

Groom's style

Flares are often only suited to tall and slim physiques, however as they would be worn with round-toe platform shoes or Cuban heels in the seventies, there is some leeway for grooms of shorter stature. Shirts tend to err on the slim-fit side and for traditional seventies style could be plain or ruffle-fronted depending on the level of formality you are after. Remember that ruffles will draw attention to ample chests and protruding stomachs so consider a plain waistcoat, which was also fashionable, if you'd rather avoid drawing attention to this area. Choose between a kipper tie, cravat or bow tie to complete your look. Hats were not considered necessary.

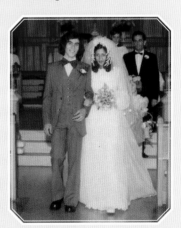

70s Checklist: Bride

Dress shape: kaftan
Dress colour: various
Dress neck: high neck
Hem length: mini to ankle length
Headdress: flower garland; Juliet cap
Shoes: platform; court

70s Checklist: Groom

Suit: single- or double-breasted; flares
Shirt: slim fit with exaggerated collars
Neckwear: cravat; tie; bow tie
Hat: none
Shoes: platforms; Cuban heels

1980s WEDDING

Bride's style

The marriage of Princess Diana to Prince Charles was the primary influence for many brides in the eighties and raised the importance of wedding gown designs to new heights. A decade obsessed with excess meant the majority of wedding dresses were made up from layers and layers of fabric with a particular emphasis on frills. The shape tends to be more fitted on the top with width on the bottom, which can be good for ladies who want to balance out a large bust. Bridal footwear favoured court shoes and sling-back sandals. With a lot of wedding dresses offering built-in support, the necessity for foundation garments will vary. However lingerie with lace details was a popular choice, with bras, suspender belts and knickers accompanied by lace-topped stockings and hold-ups.

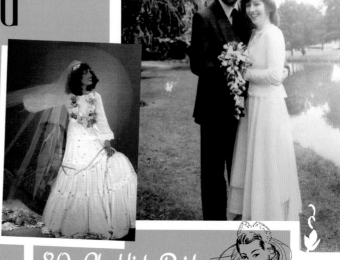

80s Checklist: Bride

Dress material & shape: lace; tiered; leg-of-mutton sleeves
Dress colour: white
Dress neck: high scoop; bateau
Hem length: mid-calf to ankle
Headdress: tiara; bows; veil
Shoes: sandals

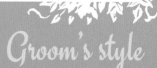

Royal Wedding

80s Checklist: Groom

Suit: single-breasted; slim leg; formal tails; waistcoat
Shirt: classic fit
Neckwear: tie or cravat
Hat: top hat
Shoes: slip-ons

Groom's style

Although out of vogue for most of the seventies, traditional groom's attire was regarded as fashionable again in the eighties, with many grooms opting for top hat and tails – a classic look appropriate for a variety of shapes and sizes. Those seeking a less ostentatious or formal approach should go for a single-breasted suit with medium-width lapels, teamed with a classic-fit shirt and tie. Slip-on shoes, particularly those with woven uppers across the bridge of the foot, will instantly add a touch of eighties class.

1990s WEDDING

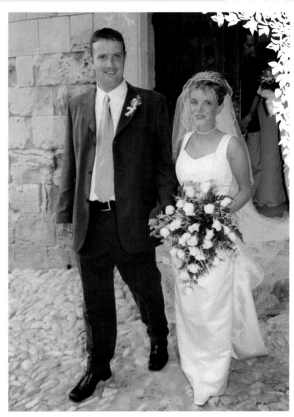

Bride's style

The 'designer' era meant that big names in haute couture fashion were creating bridal gowns for celebrities and in some cases launching entire wedding collections. Dresses moved away from frills and flounce in the 1990s, becoming much more streamlined, with shapes harking back to the twenties and thirties. With more flesh exposed in sleeveless and backless gowns and with lower necklines placing particular emphasis on the shape of the body, U-shape and multiway bras, along with tummy and hip control shorts, help create a smooth foundation. Slip-on shoes with Louis heels came back into fashion in the nineties, too.

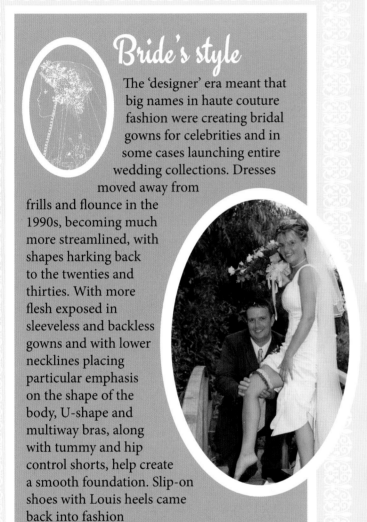

Groom's style

Having a quirky twist to the groom's attire by stepping way outside of tradition in the selection of colour palettes, patterns and design was becoming more and more popular in the nineties. In many ways, anything was acceptable and everyone was encouraged to promote their own personal style! The double-breasted suit was far less popular than the three-button single-breasted suit. However, it's best to keep the cut of the jacket classic rather than slim fit and make sure trouser legs are wide to stay true to the feel of the period. Keep in mind that the 'heroin chic' phase in fashion was brief but did influence haute couture which means that second-hand designer suits have a tendency to be cut on the extremely slim side and will not suit a large frame. Look out for vintage pieces from Paul Smith and Vivienne Westwood from this decade which often had a distinctive pattern on the outside of the garment as well as an eye-catching pattern on the inner lining. Early designs from Patrick Cox are worth looking out for, too, as he often experimented with shape as well as design. Keep shoes quite chunky with squared-off toes, buckles and a chain detail.

90s Checklist: Bride

Dress shape: fitted
Dress colour: white
Dress neck: sweetheart; square
Hem length: ankle
Headdress: tiara
Shoes: square toe; lavatory heels

90s Checklist: Groom

Suit: single-breasted; wide leg
Shirt: classic fit
Neckwear: tie
Hat: none
Shoes: chunky heels; square toes; buckles; chains

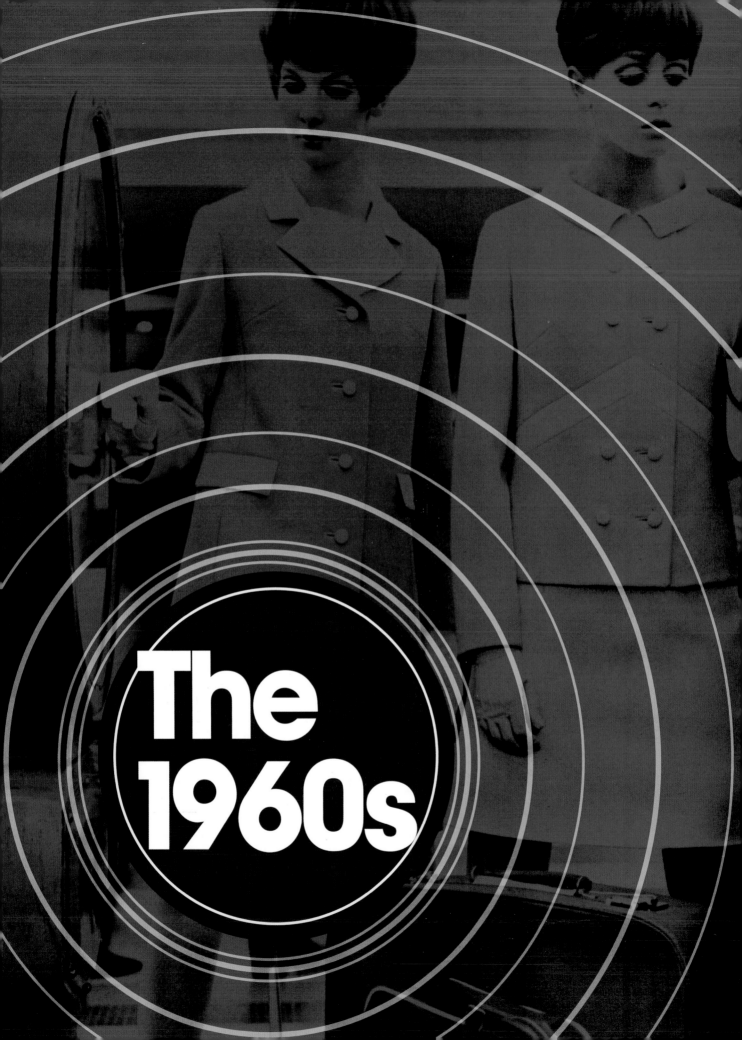

The 1960s

The sixties was a decade of dramatic contrasts. The Cuban missile crisis almost launched the world into war; America was sucked deeper into the bloody conflict in Vietnam, the Berlin Wall was built; many young people experimented with drugs and became hippies, beatniks, Rockers and Mods, and the decade ended with two astronauts walking on the Moon.

More than ever before the style of clothes that people chose to wear also became a means of showcasing their lifestyle choices, politics and attitudes. With the likes of Ossie Clark and Zandra Rhodes fresh from graduating from The Royal College of Art, it was London's turn to set the on-trend style benchmarks. A young lady by the name of Mary Quant was also in the early stages of her fashion design journey, which would shape the course of fashion for many years to come. The length of hemlines shot upwards when her designs for mini skirts and hot pants became all the rage in 'Swinging London'.

Advances in the manufacture of cosmetics and hair products meant that beauty regimes also became more dominated by the ever-changing fashions, and this would be attributed to the demise of the hat, which had been an integral part of fashion in the previous decades. Where once a lady or gentleman would not have considered leaving the house without one, the tradition of wearing a hat became passé and 'old fashioned' for the youth of the day. Sales of hairspray, hairdryer hoods and grooming equipment replaced the business that was once directed to the milliner.

Space travel was achieved, with cosmonauts Yuri Gagarin and Valentina Tereshkova blasting through the stratosphere in 1961 and 1963, sending fashion truly out of this world; Beatle-mania swept the planet as four young lads from Liverpool begged 'Love Me Do', and Martin Luther King inspired a generation to visualize a future where race held no boundaries. Catwalk models Jean Shrimpton and Twiggy became icons as they made fashion accessible to 'the girl next door'; there was also antithesis in the guise of fashion-hating 'Rockers', a group that had evolved from the 'Teds' and who wanted everything to remain just as it was in the 1950s.

Jazz was the anthem of Jean Paul Sartre-loving Beatniks who quoted writer Jack Kerouac and others from the so-called Beat Generation at the local coffee bar, whilst The Who became demi-gods to the Mods, with their love for all things Italian.

In essence, the 1960s was a time when the rule book was burnt alongside the bra, and where formal and casual dress codes were amalgamated.

1960s Women's Day Wear

Easy wear and easy care were the mantras for sixties' clothing, liberating women from the ironing board and increasing sales of clothes made from synthetic fibres. Fashion became mainstream, opening the doors to designers without formal training, such as Jean Muir, Barbara Hulanicki and Mary Quant (below left). Twiggy (right) shot to fame as a sixties supermodel, with her big eyes and ultra-petite frame suiting the new skimpy fashions. Styles were constantly changing, and fashion stores, such as Topshop and Miss Selfridge, presented new lines on a weekly basis.

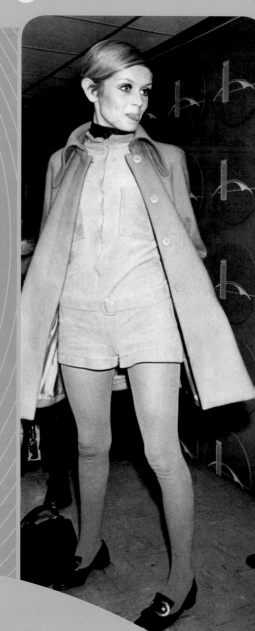

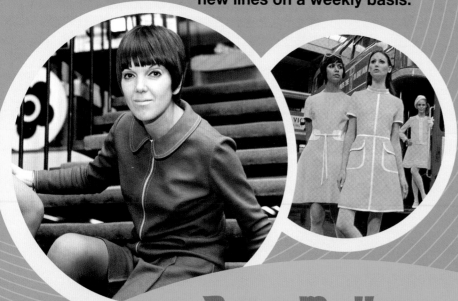

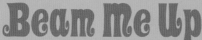

Beam Me Up

In 1969, the world's eyes were focused on the Moon after the United States landed Apollo 11 there and astronauts walked on its surface. The fascination with outer space led many designers to showcase collections that they believed would be worn in the future, with asymmetric shaping and cut-outs, and gold, silver and white featuring heavily. Many critics considered the designs just another passing fad, unlikely to be seen the following season, let alone in the future. Ironically, the clean lines and simple cuts of these 'futuristic' designs continue to be an inspiration for new designers even today.

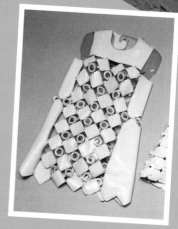

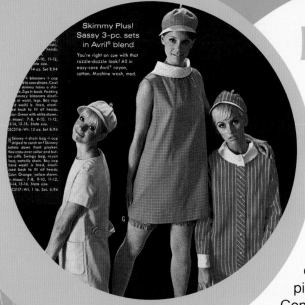

Mini v Maxi

The year 1961 gave us the Mini Cooper car and by 1964 we had the mini skirt. Although fashion had experimented with rising hem lengths a few years before, it was Mary Quant who should be credited with the responsibility of popularizing the bottom-skimming design. Many young people loved the new fashion, but some criticized the handkerchief-size pieces being marketed as clothing. Concern increased when rumours grew that wearing such tiny skirts in the winter would result in ladies developing an extra layer of fat on their thighs as the body's means of protecting itself. However, as if fashion wanted to offer an eye-pleasing solution, the all-covering maxi coat arrived.

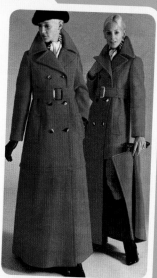

Tight Squeeze

Tights, or pantyhose, were the brain-child of a textile company CEO who was challenged by his then pregnant wife to invent something more practical than a girdle and stockings to wear with her expanding waistline. Allen Gant Sr launched 'Panti-Legs' in 1959, which combined underpants and stockings in one garment. In 1965, a seamless version was developed. This coincided with the arrival of the mini skirt and fashion followers went on to wear a variety of deniers and bright colours throughout the sixties.

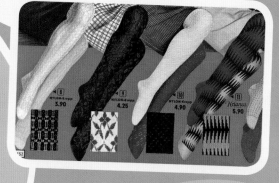

Ruffled and Frilled

With simplicity and streamlining dominating the shapes in fashion throughout the 1960s, there was a gap in the market for those yearning for ankle-grazing skirts and bygone feminine frilliness. Laura Ashley filled that opening by offering high Edwardian necklines and long smock dresses as an alternative to the flesh exposed by the majority of cutting-edge fashion. The women's wear designs of Gina Fratini and Belville Sassoon were also inspired by high romance during the decade.

Get the Look with Hannah

Choose the right hosiery to complete your sixties outfit. Go for brilliant white or strong, bold colours, such as cerise pink, orange and electric blue.

Alternative Materials

The sixties pushed fashion boundaries in almost every direction with fabrics and materials no exception. Technology was developing at warp speed and designers began to trial off-the-wall ideas. In 1966, Paco Rabanne unveiled his collection made from chainmail and plastics. Polyvinyl chloride or PVC became a staple material for everything – from boots to dresses. The fabric was widely used for raincoats throughout the decade because of its waterproof nature, but it was often criticized for being impractical as it let water in through the seams and did not allow the skin to breathe, making it quite uncomfortable to wear.

In 1966, the Scott Paper Company launched the paper dress. Obviously, paper dresses were designed to be disposable, which has made unused or carefully looked after versions, such as the 'Paper Caper' paper dress by Allendale and Abraham & Straus, highly collectable.

Art Meets Fashion

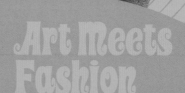

Those wanting to set trends rather than follow them were opting for wearable art. Andy Warhol, Bridget Riley and Victor Vasarely were among a wave of artists being recognized as inspirational in fashion design during the decade, with Yves Saint Laurent drawing direct inspiration from artist Piet Mondrian for his 1965 collection of the same name (left). Bold block colours, stripes and patterns were used as well as optical illusions that would trick the eye into seeing movement, a clever move for designers whose very purpose was to make people look at their creations!

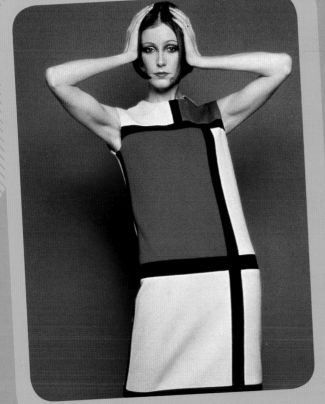

Biba Babe

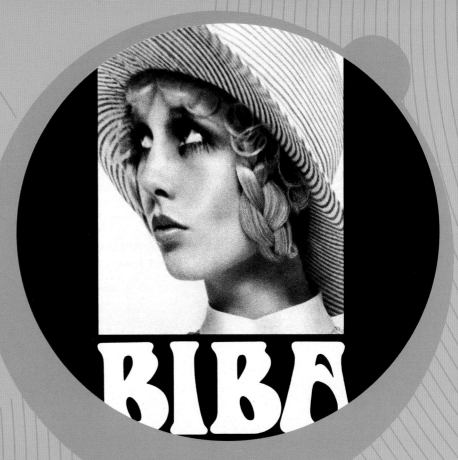

In 1963, a young Barbara Hulanicki designed a pink gingham shift dress with a key hole feature at the back and a matching kerchief which was advertised in the *Daily Mirror*. Having received 17,000 orders for that dress alone, the Biba brand was brought to Abingdon Road in Kensington, London expanding continuously until 1975. The first Biba store originally started with clothes, but it wasn't long until Biba was retailing everything from playing cards, kitchenware and make-up to pet food. Biba wasn't just a fashion label, it was a lifestyle.

The Biba brand traded on nostalgia for the past, taking elements of Art Nouveau and Art Deco which used the same lines and curves that were being seen in the psychedelic art movement as well as Victoriana and Edwardian design and combining them with a splash of the 'sixties. The trend for harking back to yesteryear was termed as retrophilia, the love of past forms. The London store was an elaborate fusion of period architecture with the trademark name in bold gold lettering on a black backdrop. Buying Biba clothes was as much about the experience of visiting the store and what celebrities you might be rubbing shoulders with as it was about the fashion being sold. Signature pieces included the smock dress and, in the later years, trousers with panel features. Colour palettes traditionally comprised berry, rust and plum tones but it was the cut of Biba garments that proved most distinctive, favouring narrow inset shoulders and tight-fitting sleeves.

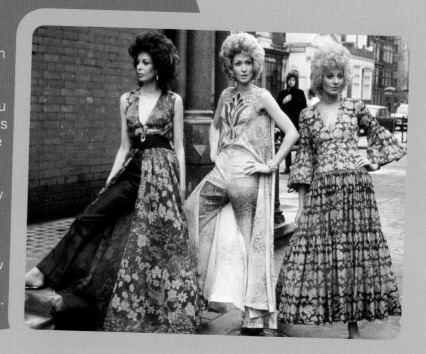

1960s Men's Day Wear

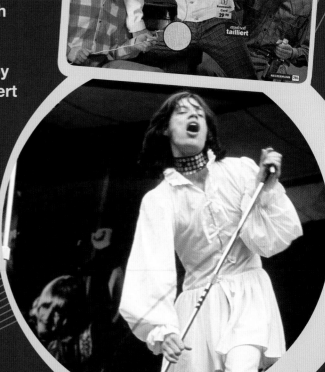

Men's wear was finally injected with more pizzazz during the sixties. Until the legalization of homosexuality in 1967, bright colours and frills had previously only been associated with gay fashion or women's wear. Fashion boundaries were pushed even further by designer Michael Fish, when in 1966 he opened his Mr Fish boutique in Mayfair – he was among the first to produce dresses for men. He famously designed a white dress worn by Mick Jagger at the Rolling Stone's concert (right) on 5th July 1969. As the decade progressed, so clothing became more unisex, and young men and women in particular found themselves shopping for outfits worn by both sexes, such as loose-fitting shirts and jeans.

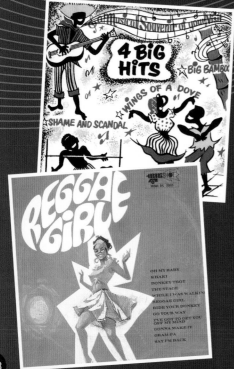

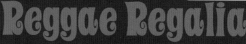

Reggae Regalia

By the mid-sixties, reggae and ska music from the Caribbean were sweeping the airwaves, and a skinhead subculture was created from a fascination with the Jamaican 'rude boy' style. This evolved to encompass drainpipe denims, checked shirts, white T-shirts, braces and large Doc Marten boots as a fashion identity. Whilst this was originally a harmless trend, it was then linked to racist political movements and became the adopted 'uniform' worn by members of the National Front in 1967. Later, it was tweaked for the punk look that developed in the following decade.

Yippee for the Hippie

Opposed to the evils of consumerism, hippies also rejected conventional values and advocated peace and love, and a love of nature. Also known as flower children, hippies wore unstructured, loose-fitting clothing, beads, bells and headbands, and both sexes generally sported long hair. The ethos of the hippie movement was to be non-conformist, and so wearing charity-shop clothes from former fashion trends offered an opportunity to indulge in a type of gentle anarchy. Many designers then started to create styles that included elements from the recent past as well from traditional 'ethnic' clothing. This resulted in the popularity of kaftan shirts in cotton or velvet, coats with mandarin collars and buckskin leather and goat-fur trim, and of long, embroidered Afghan coats.

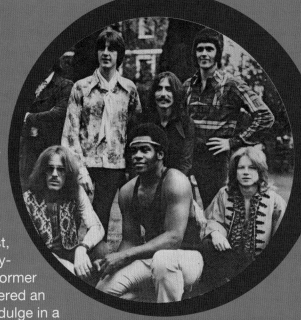

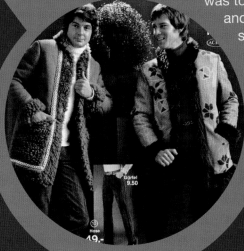

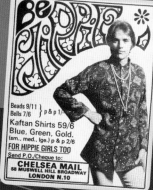

Be a HIPPIE

Beads 9/11 } p & p 1/-
Bells 7/6
Kaftan Shirts 59/6
Blue, Green, Gold.
(sm., med., lge.) p & p 2/6
FOR HIPPIE GIRLS TOO
Send P.O./Cheque to:
CHELSEA MAIL
58 MUSWELL HILL BROADWAY
LONDON N.10

Get the Look with Hannah

Incorporate some vintage style by adding a handkerchief to your breast pocket using a patterned fabric from the sixties. A lot of modern slim-fit suits can be instantly transformed with this simple twist!

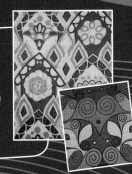

Moving to the Beat

As a Beatnik, colour choice began and ended with subtle variations of black. Fine-knit polo neck jumpers, slim-fit trousers and monochrome striped tops became part and parcel of being a beatnik, together with oversized jumpers and berets. Outer wear would most often consist of a beige double-breasted three-quarter length mac with a belted waist, which would be worn with the collar flipped up. Fiercely opposed to following any rules or convention, it was important for beatniks to express themselves intellectually rather than visually, although their 'uniform' meant their anti-fashion mandate became something of a paradox.

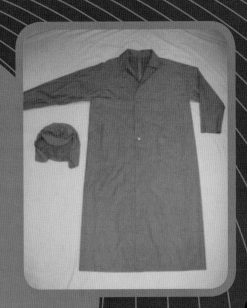

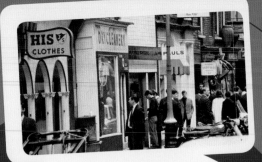

Swinging City

The 1960s have been described as 'London's decade'; fashion was increasingly defined by its youth and popular culture. Attitudes to men's wear in particular had become a lot more relaxed, with Carnaby Street the bedrock of men's fashion and a focal point for 'Swinging London'. The street drew an international audience, attracting celebrities and creating a surge in the number of boutiques, which became closely associated with the Mod and hippie sub-cultures. Merc, Lord John, Kleptomania and I Was Lord Kitchener's Valet fought for business in the heart of London's West End together with Take Six, which was based in nearby Wardour Street.

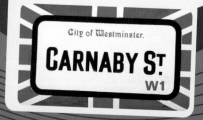

City of Westminster.
CARNABY ST.
W1

MODern Times

There is much debate over the term 'Mod' as the definition encompasses all things modern and fashionable during the decade. Some consider Mod fashion to be an extension of the beatnik style. However, the term generally conjures up an image of a tailor-made suit and parka coat, which was the outfit of choice for the young man riding a Lambretta in the sixties. Day wear and evening wear had merged to a great extent as a Mod had to look immaculate at all times. Formal jackets were mixed with casual-style trousers and were the forerunner of modern day smart-casual ensembles.

Nuts for Nutter

The cut of men's suits became increasingly sharp, with collars growing larger and longer. The slim-fit, tailored, single-breasted suit was much more in demand than the double-breasted counterpart as passion for Italian fashion grew. But it was Tommy Nutter (right) who was making a name for himself in the late sixties, bringing his style and imagination to Savile Row. Nutter combined traditional tailoring with more avant-garde designs. Nutter's signature garment was the checked blazer, but it was his willingness to experiment with fabrics and patterns, often adding a matching waistcoat, that earned him fashion notoriety.

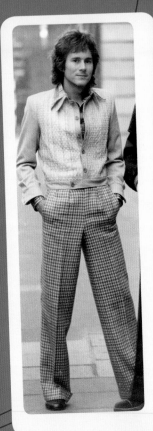

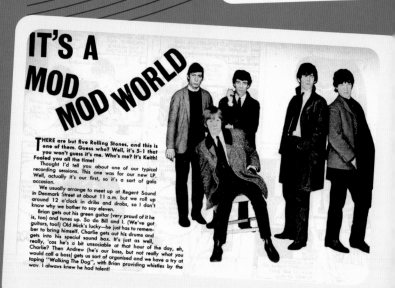

IT'S A MOD MOD WORLD

THERE are but five Rolling Stones, and this is one of them. Guess who? Well, it's 5-1 that you won't guess it's me. Who's me? It's Keith! Fooled you all the time!

Thought I'd tell you about one of our typical recording sessions. This one was for our new LP. Well, actually it's our first, so it's a sort of gala occasion.

We usually arrange to meet up at Regent Sound in Denmark Street at about 11 a.m. but we roll up around 12 o'clock in dribs and drabs, so I don't know why we bother to say eleven.

Brian gets out his green guitar (very proud of it he is, too) and tunes up. So do Bill and I. (We've got guitars, too!) Old Mick's lucky—he just has to remember to bring himself. Charlie gets out his drums and gets into his special sound box. It's just as well, really, 'cos he's a bit unsociable at that hour of the day, eh, Charlie? Then Andrew (he's our boss, but not really what you would call a boss) gets us sort of organised and we have a try at taping "Walking The Dog", with Brian providing whistles by the way. I always knew he had talent!

Loons

The ex-sailor trousers known as 'loons' became a fashion must-have for the stylish young man of the sixties. Made of cotton, loons could be striped, multicoloured or plain. They were originally made popular by a celebrity clientele, such as The Beatles and Keith Moon of The Who, among countless others. Loons started the fashion development that would become the ever popular flared torusers.

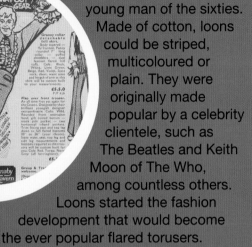

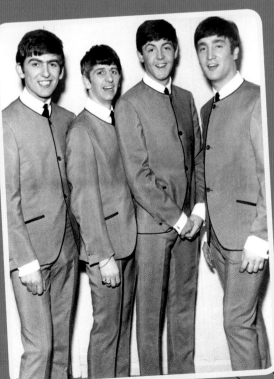

Please, Please Me

Beatlemania swept the globe during the sixties and, much like the present day, the clothing choices of the hottest band on the planet influenced millions. The Beatles' image altered considerably over time, from their early days in the fifties when John and Ringo were Teds, George an experimental follower of evolving fashion and Paul preferred a suit. They later appeared more unified when the quartet were seen sporting collarless slim-fit suits (left).

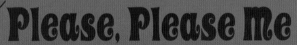

In 1960, Pierre Cardin created a five-button suit. The Nehru jacket (right) had no lapels and no trim, and was showcased to be worn done up, revealing only the smallest amount of tucked-in shirt collar or turtle-neck jumper. The trousers to go with it were narrow and straight, tapered to the ankle with no turn-ups. In 1963, Douglas Millings, the Beatles' tailor, designed an almost identical suit but with fewer buttons and black piping, which would be associated with the Fab Four for ever more.

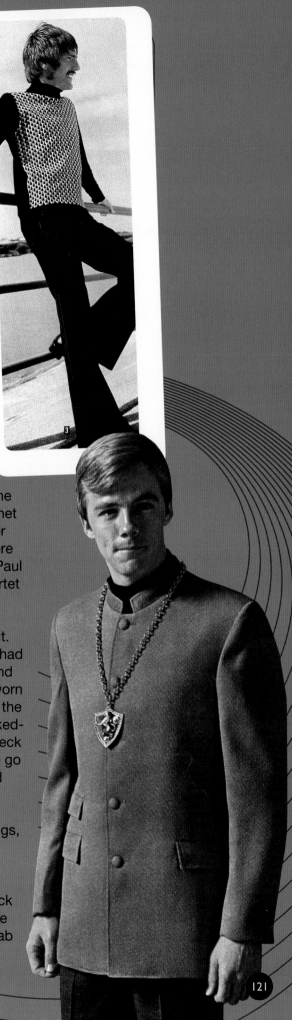

1960s Women's Evening Wear

Towards the end of the decade, evening wear had evolved to accommodate a broad spectrum of tastes, with a seemingly endless variety of length, pattern cut, fabric print and choice of embellishments. Some couturiers struggled to design glamorous gowns for the slim-line, under-developed figure that dominated fashion. Mary Quant produced designs, with baby-doll styles harking back to the flapper dresses of the twenties with their dropped waists. In contrast, Hubert de Givenchy designed his creations with a more mature audience in mind using layers, feathers and asymmetric 'necklines for a touch of drama'.

Get the Look with Hannah

Embellish a plain evening dress with feathers along the hemline for texture and shape, or diamante along the neckline for a touch of sparkle. Then embrace the fashion of the sixties completely by using the same trim on a plain envelope clutch bag for a bespoke matching accessory.

Red and White Delight

As a designer famous for his red dresses, Valentino's international debut took place in Florence in 1962. Already making waves on the fashion circuit, Valentino was deluged with orders after his collection was dubbed a fashion revelation, beginning a long association with the fashion elite. US President John Kennedy's wife, Jackie Kennedy, championed Valentino's work, famously wearing a collection of black and white dresses in the sixties as part of her year of mourning after her husband's death. The White Collection by Valentino in 1967 (right) included delicate tulle blouses, ruffled necks, organza dresses, embroidery, leather details and cashmere – all in white and ivory – and was to become possibly the most famous of his collections. Not only was it the collection that Jackie Kennedy chose for her wedding dress for her second marriage to Aristotle Onassis, but it was also the inspiration for the designer's brand signature, the 'V'.

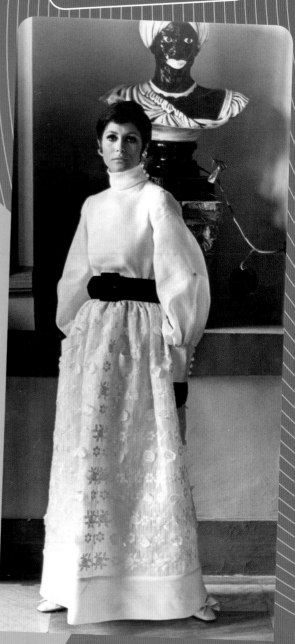

Psychedelia

As the decade progressed, the popularity of hallucinogenic drugs increased, and the textile and design industries picked up on the psychedelic trend. Designer Emilio Pucci became known for his geometric prints and kaleidoscopic colours. One of the most adored designers of the jet-set age, it is said that Marilyn Monroe was buried in one of his dresses.

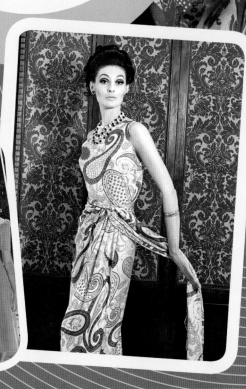

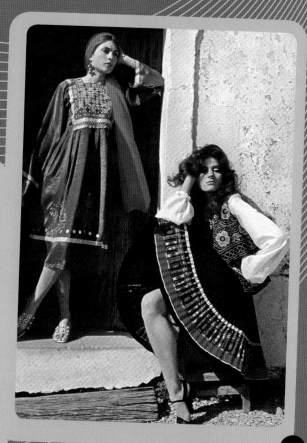

Eastern Promise

Traditional textiles and styles from Eastern countries were introduced as part of the decade's fashion trends, with Indian and Moroccan styles having a strong influence on designers' collections. Bandhani (a type of tie-dye from India) and embroidery were particularly popular, together with mirrored and fringed embellishments, creating stunningly ornate pieces worn by many of the most fashion-conscious ladies.

Zandra Rhodes cited knitting and embroidery, more specifically the chain stitch, as the inspiration for her 1969 collection – The Knitted Circle (right). The chain stitch and its variations are fundamental to the embroidery traditions of many Eastern cultures.

1960s Shoes

The footwear industry was deluged with designs in the sixties, and with mass production in overdrive, the choice was overwhelming. For women, the thin heels of the previous decades were replaced with low block heels and square toes. The days of sensible and durable fashions had gone, and with the 1960s came the 'NOW', disposable attitude. This led to the creation of footwear that simply met the demands of the latest trends with no necessity to last.

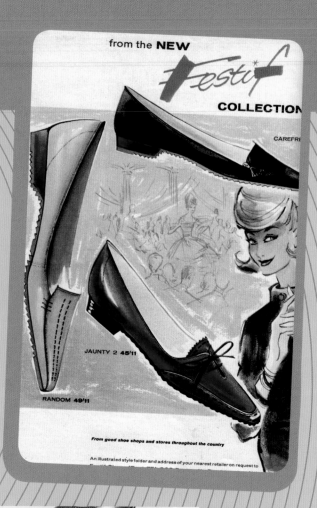

from the NEW
Festif
COLLECTION
CAREFRE

JAUNTY 2 45'11

RANDOM 49'11

From good shoe shops and stores throughout the country

An illustrated style folder and address of your nearest retailer on request to

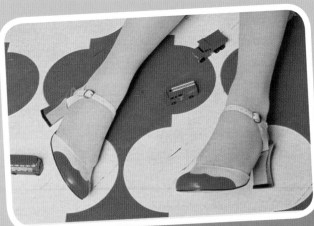

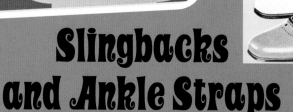

Slingbacks and Ankle Straps

Slingbacks had entered the arena of shoe design around the 1930s but proved to be a must-have fashion item in the sixties. Styles for both day and evening wear with low and high heels were created in materials that ranged from PVC and rubber to leather and exotic animal skin. Established names, such as Rayne, were moving with the changing times in order to meet the demands of society ladies. Prized for their elegant designs, Rayne enlisted the skills of Mary Quant, who was commanding the purse strings of the young and beautiful, to design her first stacked stiletto and Shirley Temple-style ankle straps for the company in 1960.

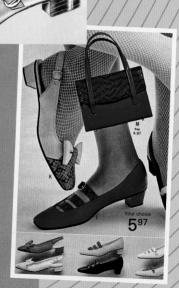

Your choice
5.97

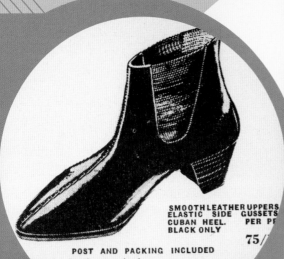

SMOOTH LEATHER UPPERS
ELASTIC SIDE GUSSETS
CUBAN HEEL. PER PR
BLACK ONLY
75/

POST AND PACKING INCLUDED
on the Continent only for—

RONA LTD., 1 HALLSWELLE PARA
LONDON N.W.11

FROM THE ABOVE

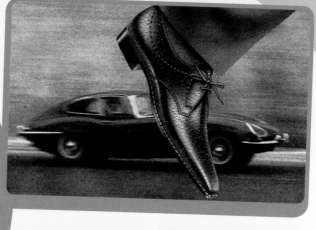

Chelsea Boots

Unisex Chelsea boots became an integral part of the footwear associated with the Mods and therefore an iconic item of 1960's fashion. Sometimes referred to as the Beatle Boot (after Cuban heel versions were commissioned by Lennon and McCartney from Anello & Davide in the 1960s), and demand for the style increased. The boots were available in a wide variety of materials, including leather and suede, and in some cases PVC. They all required the assistance of a strong shoe horn as the tightly bound elasticated sides meant the boots were often extremely difficult to get on.

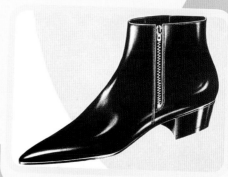

Boots

Boots worn with short skirts became a real fashion statement during the decade. In 1966, Nancy Sinatra released a record that made the humble boot the centre of attention. 'These Boots Are Made For Walking' reached No. 1 in America in February 1966. Then, when Jane Fonda emerged as a futuristic bombshell in thigh-high white PVC boots in the movie *Barbarella (left)* in 1968, she almost instantly changed the way the footwear was viewed. The utilitarian boot was elevated from being functional fashion to sultry and sexy and set the precedent for over-the-knee and thigh-high boots in mainstream fashion.

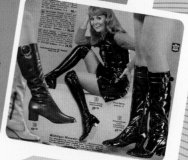

125

1960s Sportswear

After the television programme *Match of The Day* was first broadcast in 1964, it wasn't long before the TV channels gave into public pressure for regular televised coverage of other sports. The programme *World of Sport* was launched in 1965, and this fuelled an increase in the demand for a wide variety of leisurewear options in the UK. The popularity of sport and awareness of the benefits of fitness meant that tracksuits, although worn by professional athletes 'track side', were ideal attire for the regular man and woman engaging in general sports. Adidas branched out to include this apparel in 1961 with its first range, the Adidas Schwahn tracksuit, which became an instant success.

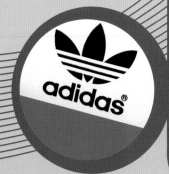

Boxing Clever

The Lonsdale brand hit the West End of London when ex-boxer Bernard Hart launched his company in 1960. Located in Soho's Beak Street, initially Lonsdale sold only boxing equipment but being in such close vicinity to Carnaby Street meant the store rapidly expanded into selling fashionable sportswear that was worn by pop and film stars alike. Boxing reached dizzying heights of popularity when Henry Cooper fought Muhammad Ali at Wembley Stadium in 1963.

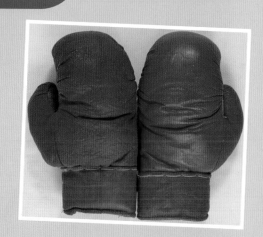

They Think It's All Over...

In 1966 sportswear was introduced to a new global audience when England lifted the football World Cup, having defeated Germany in a tense final. Umbro had signed a deal to supply the England team's kit, which comprised a plain white, long-sleeved, round-neck top with a badge showing three small lions on the left breast, and black shorts. However, because Germany also played in the same colours, there had to be a coin toss to see which country would wear their choice of kit. England lost and, as a result, had to play the final in their alternative strip of red tops with white hsorts and red socks. However, this immediately made that football strip a piece of fashion history and Umbro is still producing replica red kits to the present day.

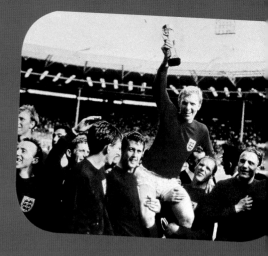

Bowled over!

The craze for tenpin bowling in the United States spread to the UK in the sixties. The unisex-style, loose-fit shirts and round-toe tie-up shoes worn to play the sport were eagerly purchased but the trend was short-lived and had all but died out by the mid-seventies.

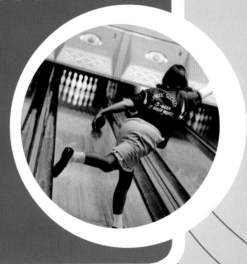

Get the Look with Hannah

Vintage sports bags add a retro feel to an outfit, with brands such as Slazenger, Adidas, Lonsdale and Dunlop being quite collectable. Check the handles and straps for cracks and tears as you may need to consider the cost and practicality of repairs.

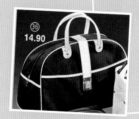

Speedy Feet

Sports footwear experienced a lot of technical advances in the 1960s, when manufacturers finally realized that a sports shoe was more than just something that had to look good. The first sports shoes (sneakers) failed to offer the wearer much support and provided no buffer to any impact or wear on the joints when worn for sports. They caused runners excessive shin splints and, as more and more people took up different sporting activites, so the materials that were used and the technical design evolved. In 1961, The Trackster by New Balance was one of the first shoes to be designed specifically for running.

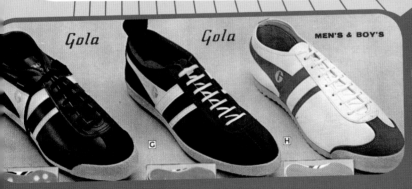

Gola   Gola   MEN'S & BOY'S

1960s Accessories

The frequent changes in fashion in the decade created, meant an abundance of choice. Accessories were no exception and it was possible to mix and match handbags, ties, handkerchiefs, jewellery, hats, sunglasses and more to complement an ever-changing, disposable wardrobe. Some designs have stood the test of time and remained a fashion staple to the present day, with bold colours, plastic and metal featuring heavily as well as 'pop art' and 'op art' designs.

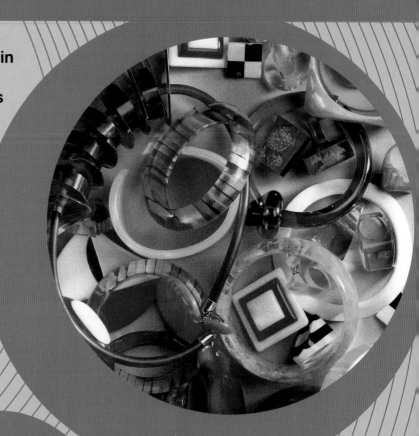

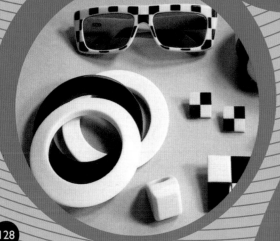

Those favouring quality over quantity continued to wear fine jewellery over costume pieces. However, cutting-edge designers such as Lanvin, Courrèges and Rabanne seized the opportunity to offer the latest accessories to complement their collections.

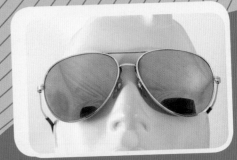

In the Shades

Sunglasses had become a fashion accessory some two decades earlier but the overriding design of the sixties was the 'Aviator'. Originally designed by Ray-Ban in the thirties, the unisex mirrored design reigned, and has held its place in the fashion world until the present day.

Sweet Smell of Success

Men wore fresh, citrusy *Eau Sauvage* (1966) by Dior or *Bay Rhum* by Royall (1962), containing bay leaf, green grass and mint. Fabergé's *Brut* and *Brut 33* were definitely an acquired taste, but probably the best-known fragrance of the decade was Pfizer's *Hai Karate*. A forerunner of *Lynx*, it was sold with a self-defence manual to ward off uncontrollable women! It was launched in 1967 and attracted a lot of attention as a result of its clever marketing, and became a popular box set for boyfriends and husbands. Although *Hai Karate* is no longer manufactured, it can still be obtained and remains a really evocative reminder of a bygone era. Popular women's perfumes included *Oh! De London* (1962) by Tuvaché, *Rose* by Molinard (1960) and *Calèche* by Hermès (1961), which all contained strong floral notes.

Get the Look with Hannah

Although mass production was big in the sixties, investing in quality pieces will almost always ensure longevity. Look out for named items of jewellery. Companies like Weiss, Sarah Coventry, Coro and Trifari created some beautiful designs, as did Whiting & Davis, which launched a 'Cleopatra' collection in 1963 to tie in with the Elizabeth Taylor movie of the same name.

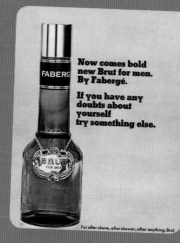

Now comes bold new Brut for men. By Fabergé.

If you have any doubts about yourself try something else.

For after shave, after shower, after anything. Brut.

Cool Cravats

Cravats were a really simple fashion accessory which became a popular choice for both sexes in the sixties and beyond. Both men and women (who were increasingly embracing opportunites to wear trouser suits) would accompany their look with bold, bright patterns which, in some instances, would be an exact match with their shirt or blouse. Emilio Pucci seized upon this trend, launching a wide range of classic Pucci print silk ties, which was a huge success.

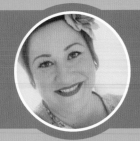

1960s Get the Look with Hannah

The sixties were full of bold colour. Key shades from the early years were reminiscent of those from the fifties (pastels as well as reds, blues and greens). However, as the decade progressed there were lots of vivid yellows, cerise pinks, day-glo oranges and lime greens, so play around with different colours to see what looks good. For make-up, colour choice depended on age group. Younger women went for monochrome eye colours and nude lip tones, while more mature ladies favoured lilac and blue hues with magenta and pink lip shades.

Big Hips

DO
...wear shift dresses and wide loon pants as these can create balance.

DON'T
...wear ultra-short mini skirts or dresses as these can be unflattering.

Large Bust

DO
....opt for a V-neck to create balance.

DON'T
....wear high collars or polo necks as these will only emphasize a large bust.

Petite

DO
....try a beehive hairdo to create volume and height
....consider the pixie hair cut.

DON'T....be afraid to wear maxi coats; just ensure they are altered to suit your height.

Men

Men's hairstyles were influenced by war and music with the crew cut, Ivy League crew cut and the layered shag dominant both in the US and UK, while women embraced big, long and groomed-to-perfection hair.

Tall

DO
....wear minI skirts and shift dresses to show off those pins!
....wear intricate patterns.
....wear maxi coats.

DON'T
....be afraid to wear heels.
....wear all-over bold block. patterns

Naturally Straight Hair

DO
....consider 'cheating' a short hairstyle by pinning up long hair.

DON'T
....forget to use an appropriate hair product to achieve curls or flicks.

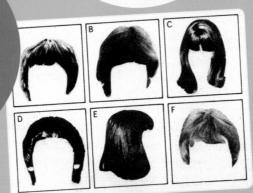

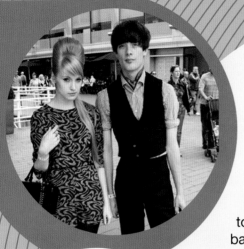

BIG HAIR

Making the most of hair was all the rage, and beehives were very popular. But not all hair types can achieve this style. Backcombing fine or dry hair can be damaging, and achieving long-lasting flick-ups can be impossible for those with poker-straight hair, so always consider your hair type before trying to create a particular look. If you have established that backcombing wiil work for your hair, follow these rules: backcomb from the root and use scooping motions and broad strokes – you don't want to end up with a tangled mess! Use an appropriate product such as mousse or root lift and ensure you have plenty of lacquer for a firm hold. If you are using heat appliances like hair tongs or straighteners to achieve shape, use a heat spray first to protect the hair.

The sharp bob sported by Mary Quant is best attempted by those with straight hair as the style is in the sleek silhouette it creates.

AFRO!

Afro hair was worn with pride and combed into magnificent heights. To achieve the perfect sixties afro, invest in a shampoo and conditioner that have the right balance of protein and moisturizer so your hair does not become dry and brittle. Buy a large paddle brush, wide-tooth comb/pick and a hair product to reduce tangles.

Never brush dry hair. Spritz through water and oil or a tangle-minimizing product and divide hair into sections (the thicker your hair, the more sections you need).

Take each section, start at the tip and use the paddle brush to brush through the hair to the root.

For short to mid-length hair, rub styling wax between your palms and gently pat your afro all around, creating the perfect circle shape.

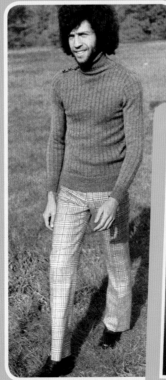

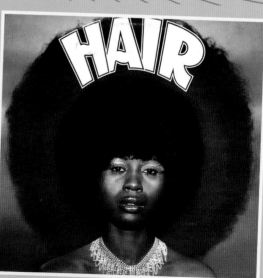

ASK THE EXPERT

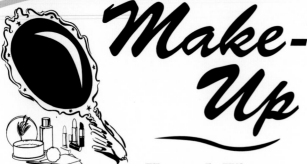

Make-Up

***Hannah Wing** is a make-up artist, author and stylist. She was given a 1920s Lucite compact as a gift and that was the start of her obsession with vintage make-up and beauty products. As a self-confessed vintage addict, she has amassed numerous collections over the years, with a particular interest in retro make-up and beauty ephemera.*

What types of make-up do you like to collect?

All sorts! I don't limit myself simply to make-up – I also collect beauty- and hair-related items, so everything from hairdryers, hair tongs and compacts

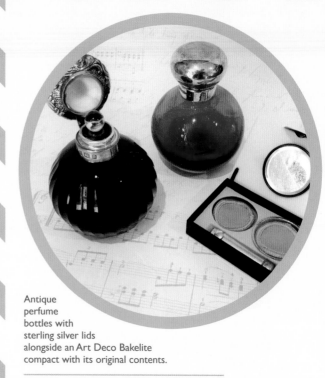

Antique perfume bottles with sterling silver lids alongside an Art Deco Bakelite compact with its original contents.

to lipsticks, cold creams and perfumes. It's usually the packaging that catches my eye especially if it evokes the essence of the period in which it was produced.

What's the best way to preserve vintage make-up?

It's best to keep make-up at room temperature and to make sure it's not placed in direct sunlight.

Where do you go to buy items to add to your collection?

I'm always on the lookout, so car boot sales, garage sales, charity shops, church and school fetes and vintage emporiums. Lots of friends know I collect so they keep an eye out, too.

Is vintage make-up easy to collect?

Real vintage make-up and beauty tools in good condition are actually quite rare as they weren't designed to last 50 or 100 years. Perfume bottles and compacts tend to be easier to come across.

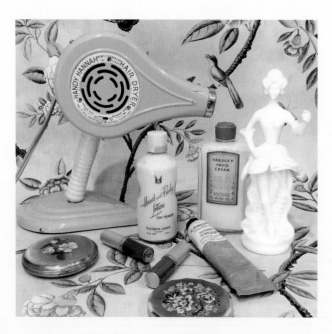

Handy Hannah hairdryer (circa 1950), hand and body lotions from Elizabeth Arden and Yardley from the same period and an Avon *Moonwind* perfume bottle from 1971.

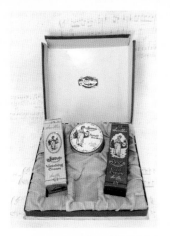
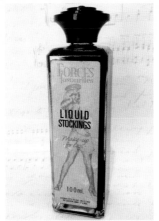

A 1920s Saville's June toiletry set complete with cold cream, beauty powder and vanishing cream in original box (left). Forces Favourite 1940s style liquid stockings (circa 1990, right).

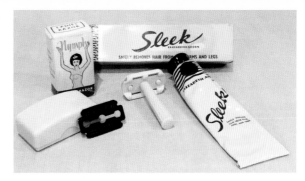

Nymph travel razor and sleek hair removal cream (circa 1950).

Is vintage make-up expensive?

It varies dramatically. Vintage make-up can be picked up really cheaply but tools, compacts and perfume prices can go into thousands of pounds depending on the age, rarity and materials used. Some compacts are made from platinum, gold or sterling silver and might be embellished with diamonds or other precious stones so obviously these can cost a small fortune. Even some early perfumes that were produced in limited editions were packaged in cases that are considered works of art in their own right.

Are there any particular names or designs to look out for?

Cartier, Van Cleef & Arpels, Fabergé, and Tiffany are some of the more exclusive names; however, sterling silver or solid gold compacts with enamel are also highly collectable. At the more reasonable end of the scale, Estée Lauder have been producing collectable compacts for many years as well as collectable solid perfumes. I have a few that were made in conjunction with Strongwater, which are gorgeous.

Do you have any tips for what not to buy?

Avoid badly damaged compacts that have a broken mirror or large chips out of the enamel. These will devalue the item considerably. Avoid buying items in containers that are cracked or broken as these will inevitably leak and could ruin other items in your collection.

Should collectors keep or remove powder in vintage compacts or perfume in vintage bottles?

No! Whilst I wouldn't advocate using vintage make-up on the skin, if the compact has been stored correctly, the powder will do no harm. If hand-pressed powder has been broken and is likely to create a mess, then discard it. Perfume is quite different, depending on the concentration. Some mixes are 33 per cent or 60 per cent perfume oil or, in some herb-based fragrances like lavender, 100 per cent. The higher the purity of the oil, the more likely it is not to have spoilt. If a perfume has gone off, chances are you will notice a darkening of the liquid (in a see-through bottle) but if you can't tell by looking, simply give it a sniff – you'll soon know!

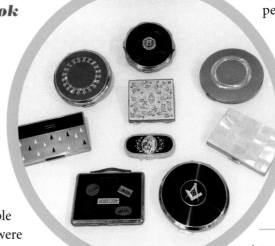

A small selection of vintage compact mirrors from manufacturers including Kigu, Stratton, Coty and Estée Lauder.

133

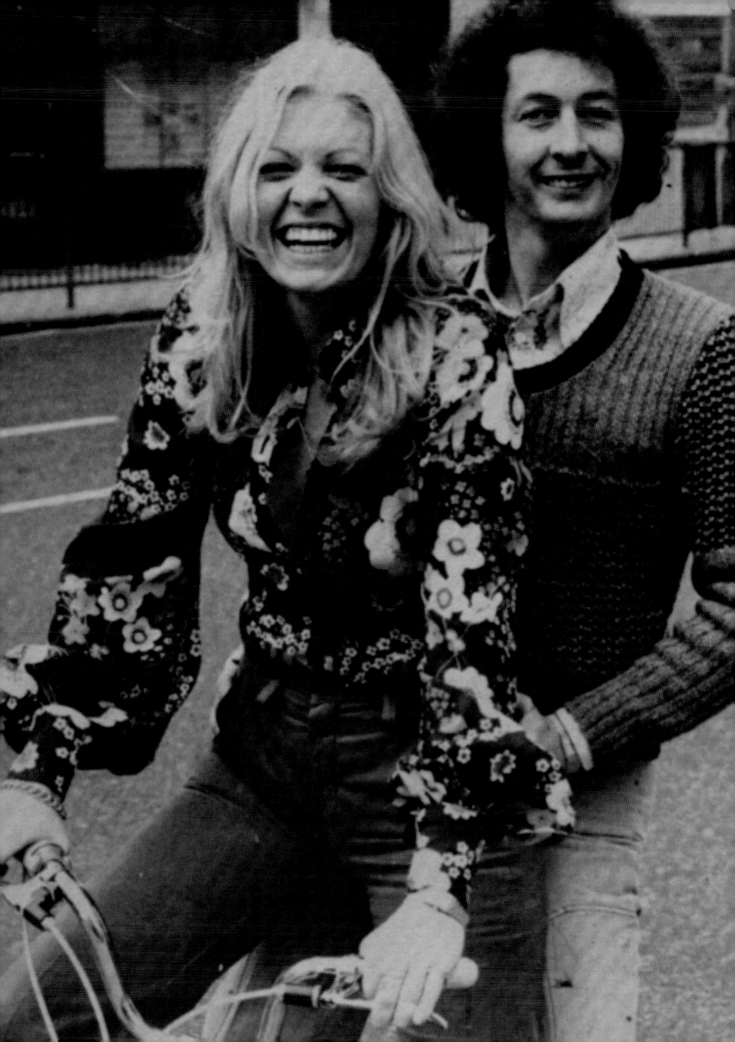

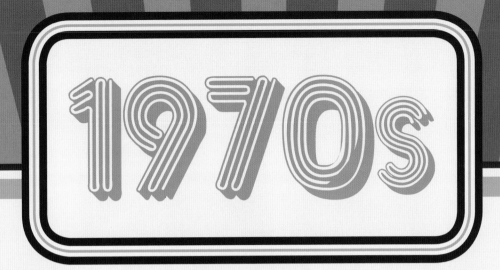

1970s

For the most part, men and women of the seventies had moved on from the newness and excitement of the sexual liberation of the sixties, with the majority of consumers preferring to opt for a more subdued and relaxed fashion style. This was, of course, with the exception of those with a more aggressive and subversive approach to their attire – the punks.

At the beginning of the decade the fashion colour spectrum was vast but the overriding preference was for more subdued colours, and the earthy hues of browns, yellows and oranges were favoured. This was a time when many people sought to get back to nature, when outfits were simplified to suit both the male and female form, and when layering and unisex clothing really came to the forefront of fashion.

Against the background of the Vietnam War, the three-day week and the introduction of decimalization in Britain, the seventies saw massive political unrest. Fashion turned to the ideology of harmony, peace and tolerance. Designers embraced ideas from foreign cultures, diverse religions and ethnic influences and brought these into the British and American mainstream. Beverley Johnson was the first black model to appear on the front of American *Vogue* in August 1974 and influential fashions were modelled by exotic beauties such as Donyale Luna and Talitha Getty. But then substance abuse claimed both their lives in the early seventies and the likes of Marisa Berenson, Veruschka and Lauren Hutton, with their clear skin, minimal make-up and Amazonian physiques, set the trend for a healthy lifestyle and became the role models of many young women.

Hemlines yo-yoed, sleeves and side seams expanded and contracted rapidly, necklines became asymmetrical and 'vintage style' dress was seen on the catwalk. By the late seventies, fashion was starting to be influenced by the concepts of power, excess and rebellion, which shaped the stage for the dawn of the next decade.

1970s WOMEN'S DAY WEAR

Much of women's fashion from the early part of the decade veered too far on the 'conservative' spectrum for some. The long hemlines on skirts and dresses being showcased by top designers were perceived by some to incite the repression of women. This resulted in public protests on the streets of New York City. However, it was actually a direct response to demands for more universally 'wearable' dresses and skirts as an alternative to mini skirts, which were only being worn by the young and super slim. In sharp contrast, lacy necklines and cuffs became part of mainstream fashion in the seventies. The trend for ruffles and romance and Victorian and Edwardian-inspired styling saw the further rise in popularity of Welsh fashion designer Laura Ashley, who had expanded her clothing range.

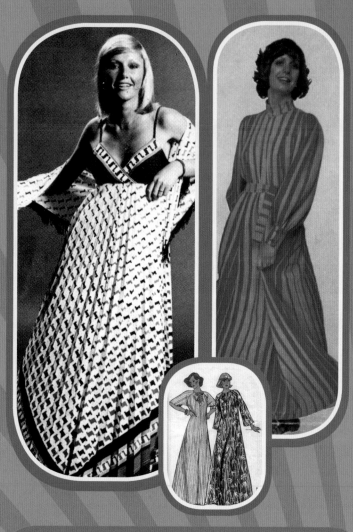

Wartime Revival

Former fashion styles weren't just being sported by hippies who dressed from charity shops – it was a growing trend amongst couturiers, too. Many designers injected 1940s style into 1970s collections with their take on siren suits, featuring wide lapels and gathered shoulders, and tea dresses in miniature floral patterns. This trend included designer of the moment Yves Saint Laurent with his Liberation collection from 1971, which was inspired by the style of his French-Algerian mother and that of close friend French fashion designer Paloma Picasso, who had a penchant for vintage silk dresses and Bakelite jewellery.

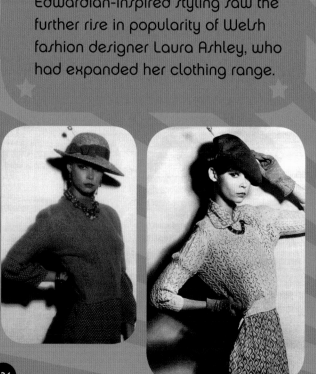

Boho Chic

The kaftan was the epitome of unstructured garments and became hugely popular during the decade. Roy Halston Frowick, best known simply as 'Halston', was the godfather of simplicity in his designs, receiving much acclaim for his use of synthetic suede leather, which became known as ultrasuede. Brought into the fashion arena in the late sixties, the floor-length skirt and dress became part of the seventies 'look'. It embraced every shape and size, hiding a multitude of sins and creating body-size 'freedom', something not often embraced by the fashion industry.

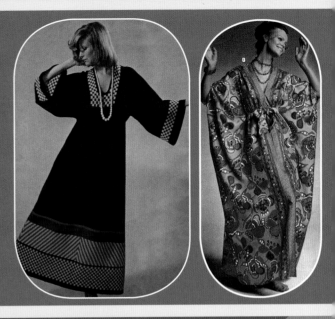

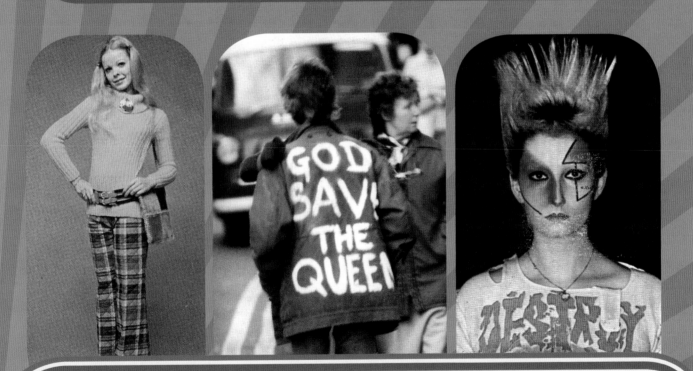

Sound Waves

Fashion and music had been influencing one another since the early fifties. The diversity that had evolved over the years meant that audiences made choices based as much on a singer's or a band's image as they did their music. Groups such as Slade, Roxy Music and the Bay City Rollers

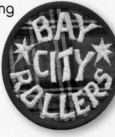

and singers such as David Bowie commanded huge followings in the seventies, sparking epic explosions of tartan and 'alternative' apparel. The Dammed, The Clash and The Sex Pistols represented the anti-establishment ethos of the punk movement. Punks cut up clothes from charity shops and held them together with safety pins and chains. Hair was worn spiked in a Mohican style.

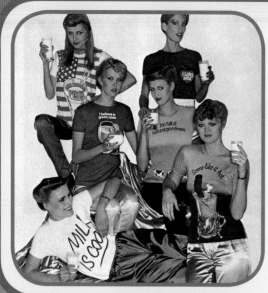

Tee-total

Photographs of topless models appeared regularly on page 3 of a British newspaper for the first time in the 1970s, This took away much of the taboo around staring at women's breasts, and as women realized they had assets they could flaunt designers realized they could showcase these assets to their own advantage. The slogan T-shirt developed into a staple for fashion designers and became a piece of marketing gold. For the first time in fashion history, it wasn't the cut of the clothes alone that confirmed a designer's signature, it was the slogan and brand advertising positioned across the chest.

Get the Look with Hannah

Ponchos, gauchos and capes became the outer wear extension to the free-flowing fashion of the period. They allow layering, which makes them perfect for wearing all year round. And crochet capes look great over bikinis on the beach.

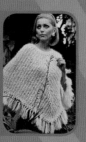

Sex

Politically charged, sexually experimental and highly rebellious, Vivienne Westwood and her partner Malcolm McLaren introduced the Kings Road to their shop SEX in 1971. Initially selling extreme bondage wear for both men and women, the pair later changed the shop name from SEX to Seditionaries in 1976, selling a range of so-called 'anti-fashion' – customized denim, ripped T-shirts held together with safety pins, pink plastic biker jackets and tartan drill, which were labelled 'trash' by the critics. This did nothing to stop the success of their collections, as punk subculture swelled and Westwood went on to become one of the most celebrated and collected fashion designers of all time.

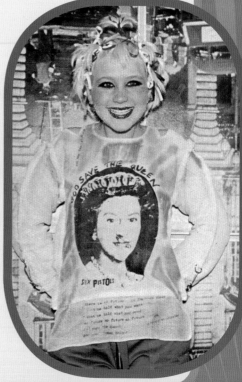

Crochet Capers

Crochet was used in all aspects of fashion and accessories in the seventies in men's, women's and children's ranges as well as homeware.

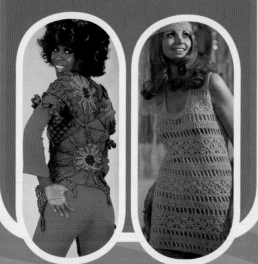

Native New Yorker

Many fashion designers adopted timeless, easy-to-wear styles in the 1970s to suit women's natural figures. This prompted designer Calvin Klein to define a New York aesthetic. With a range of interchangeable separates, Klein appealed to the expanding female professional workforce with his use of luxury fabrics and classic styling.

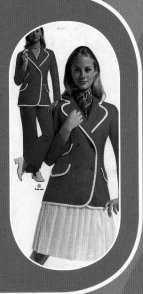

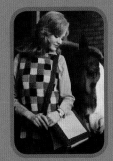
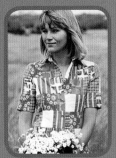

Patch & Quilt

Throughout the decade the trend for customizing and upcycling clothes grew beyond hippy circles. Both quilting and patchwork were used extensively, especially on coats, jumpers and dresses.

Skinny Ribs

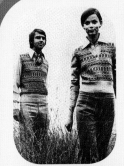

Skinny-rib, tight-fitting jumpers and tank tops with wide scoop or high polo necks were commonly worn with hipster flares.

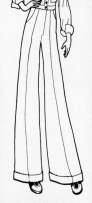

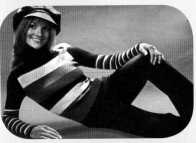

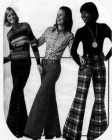

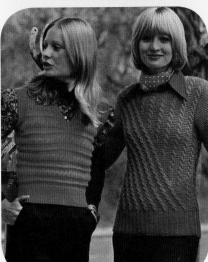

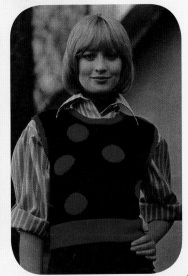

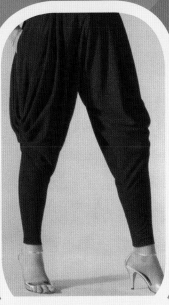

Pants Power

Women had worn trousers for decades but they weren't generally accepted as feminine or fashionable until the seventies. Harem pants were introduced in 1913 by French designer Paul Poiret. His loose-fitting, wide-leg design was the inspiration for parachute pants and palazzo pants, which became popular with women.

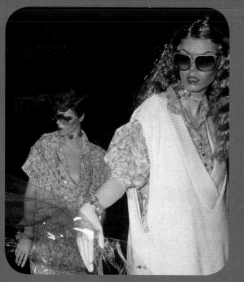

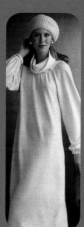

The Big Look

The 'big look', or 'the droop' as it was otherwise known, was introduced to fashion in 1974. The figure-hugging designs popular in the early years of the decade were overtaken by the trend for raglan sleeves and oversizing. Big look clothes 'drooped' off of small frames and gave meaning to the idea that 'one size fits all'.

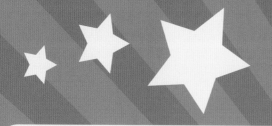

Nautical but Nice

Naval uniforms and all things nautical crept into fashion in the seventies. This trend created a surge in yachting motifs and flared sailor suits on the fashion catwalks.

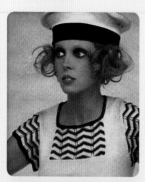

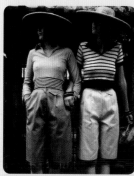

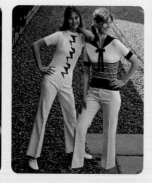

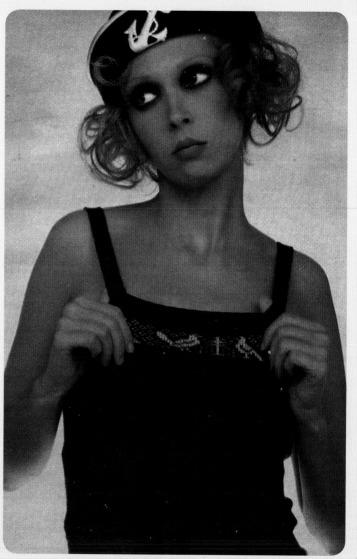

Flashing Hazards

Television played a huge role in popularizing fashion trends for both men and women. A popular American TV series of the period was *The Dukes of Hazard*, which gave us 'Daisy Duke' with her penchant for cut-off denim shorts. These became a day time version of hot pants, typically worn with a checked shirt tied in a knot under the bust, exposing the midriff.

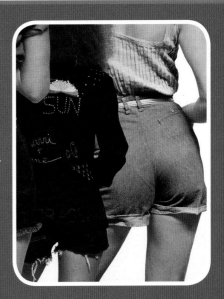

Jumping for Joy

The jump suit was both functional and stylish, offering the best of both worlds. Although the all-in-one concept had been seen as long ago as the forties with the wartime siren suit, the flared legs, pockets, zip front and cuff sleeves had a definite seventies slant.

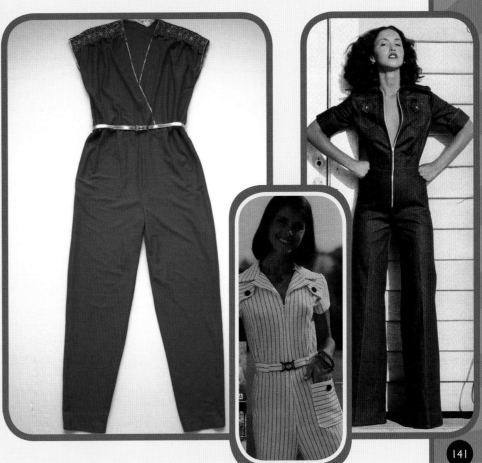

1970s MEN'S DAY WEAR

The 1970s man embraced soft fashion designs and materials previously reserved for women's wear. This was almost a natural evolution as unisex fashion became more acceptable and saw men's wear ranges with belted waists and materials, such as faux fur being used for coats. Many men adopted a broader colour palette too, as lighter, previously considered feminine shades were incorporated into day and evening wear. This not only helped expand the boundaries of design concepts for men's collections, but also paved the way for the gender-neutral fashion trends of the future.

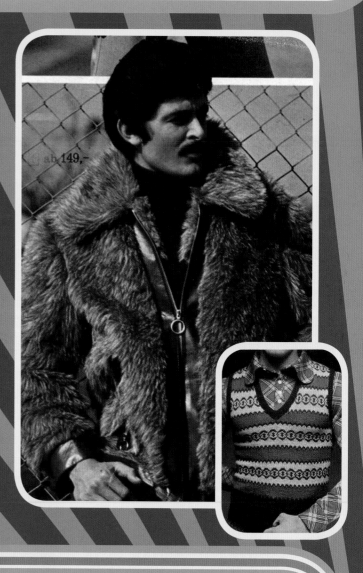

Polo Match

Ralph Lauren began his career in the sixties, designing men's neckties under his Polo label. In 1970, he was given the Coty Award for his menswear designs, an accolade that inspired him to expand into women's wear. In 1972 he made a bold move to release a men's short-sleeve cotton shirt in no less than 24 different colours, all emblazoned with the Polo logo, which would become the signature look for his brand.

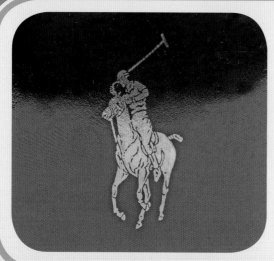

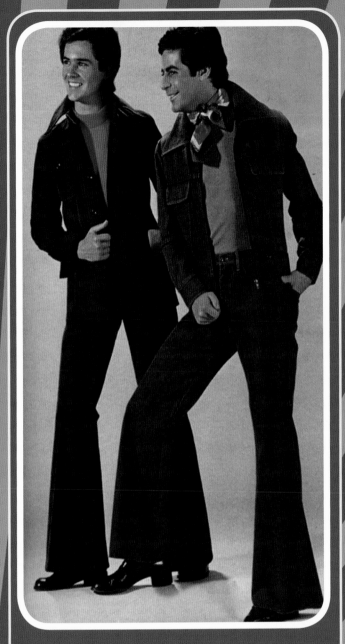

Y-not?

As women's clothing seemed to get baggier, menswear moved to the other end of the spectrum, making it necessary to ditch loose-fitting underwear in favour of Y-fronts. This supportive undergarment was first introduced in 1935 and divided audiences. Some loved the appendage-hugging apparel, while others continued to wear looser underwear and trousers, which they felt were more modest!

Denim Delights

Jacob Davis and Levi Strauss invented blue jeans in 1873, which 100 years later had become a wardrobe staple for men and women. The prevailing style during the decade was mid to high waist with a boot-cut base, although hippies wore enormous flared versions. Many personalized their jeans by adding rhinestones or deliberately ripped them for a distressed look. Patched denim was also popular, and styles varied between just a few patches to an entire pair made from bold squares of dyed denim.

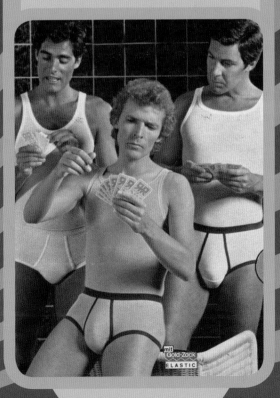

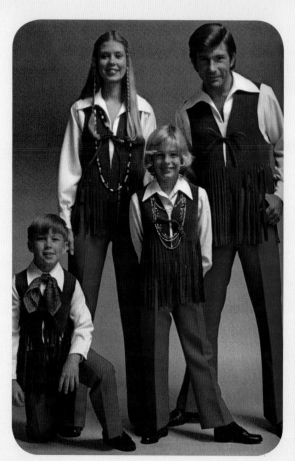

A Family Affair

When celebrities David and Victoria Beckham were photographed in matching outfits it created much chatter in fashion circles although it wasn't a new concept. Unisex fashion was all the rage and this gave way to a trend for uniformity that galvanized the 'his and hers' look and took it one step further to extend clothing ranges to the whole family!

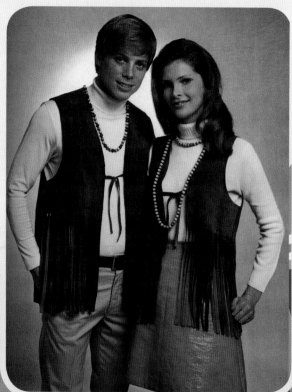

Giorgio Armani

Giorgio Armani launched his designs in July 1975 with a men's clothing line with no excess detail and using simple textiles. He also added a colour to the otherwise brown, yellow and orange spectrum of the day, calling it 'greige' – a fusion of grey and beige that resulted in a light oatmeal colour.

Get the Look with Hannah

Dungarees were a popular fashion choice in the seventies, and they can be both stylish and practical to wear. Ladies should team a pair of mid-blue denim flared dungarees with a spaghetti-strap striped vest and slip on some platform wedges for a classic period look. Make sure you accessorize with a fringed cross-body bag and lots of bangles.

On Safari

Unisex fashion grew throughout the period with Rudi Gernreich, Ted Lapidus and Yves Saint Laurent bringing the concept into haute couture. The re-emergence of the *safari suit* was one such creation, which made its mark in warmer climates, especially Australia. The classic safari jacket was made in a lightweight material. It was self-belting and had expanding bellows pockets with popper fastenings. The trousers matched in colour and material, and were a loose fit with a slight flare at the hem. This style has remained a classic moving in and out of mainstream fashion since its first appearance as casual wear in the early 1950s.

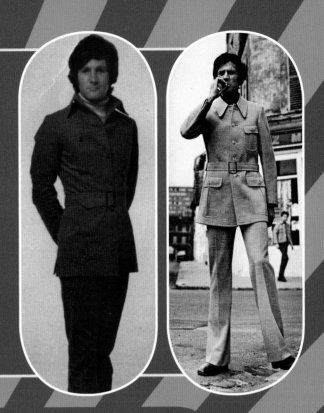

Knit Wit

Single-colour polo necks, bold knitted vests and jumpers with patterns were all the rage for men. Knitwear had become much chunkier by the 1970s and oversize cardigans were made 'cool' by the likes of actor Paul Michael Glaser's character in the popular television programme, *Starsky & Hutch*.

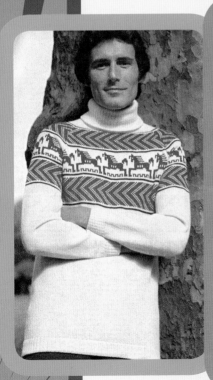
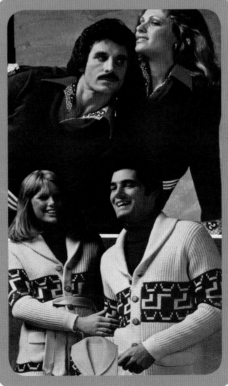
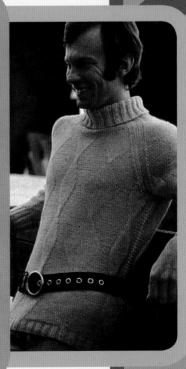

145

1970s WOMEN'S EVENING WEAR

Not since the 1920s had ladies shimmered and sparkled quite so much in their evening attire. From the dance floors of Studio 54 in Manhattan to the Embassy Club in London, disco balls were reflecting the light of a million sequins. There was an increasing influx of both Japanese style and designers, with the Far East fast putting 'quirky' into the mix, with names like Kenzo Takada and Kansai Yamamoto showcasing collections inspired by geisha kimonos and kabuki theatre. Fashion was intrinsically linked to music and singers and musicians often influenced fashion trends. Fashion couple Ossie Clark and Celia Birtwell even lived with rock guitar legend Jimi Hendrix. for a time.

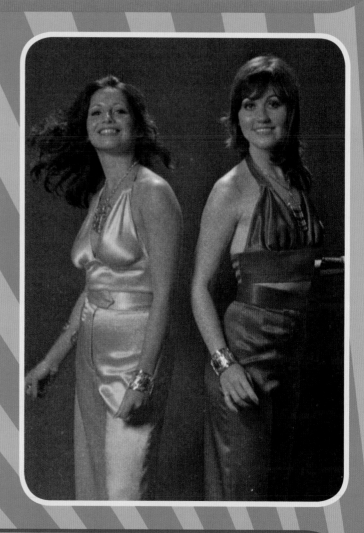

Boogie Nights

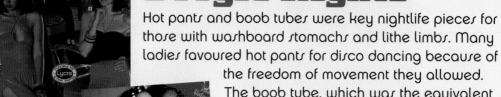

Hot pants and boob tubes were key nightlife pieces for those with washboard stomachs and lithe limbs. Many ladies favoured hot pants for disco dancing because of the freedom of movement they allowed. The boob tube, which was the equivalent design for the top half of the body, claimed to have been popularized by Israeli-American designer Elie Tahari in 1971. Boob tubes were made from elasticated fabric and were often embellished with sequins that would reflect the lights on the disco dance floor.

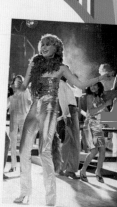

Vintage Revival

Although 1940's Hollywood glamour was predominant in seventies designs, American fashion designer Halston championed 1930s backless evening gowns, teamed with deep plunging necklines and asymmetric necklines that exposed a single shoulder. Elsa Schiaparelli had used these neckline styles as a feature on many of her Grecian dresses in the thirties and provided the inspiration for the coveted Halston gowns.

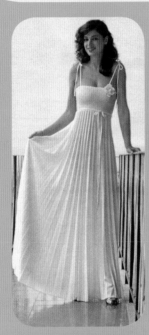

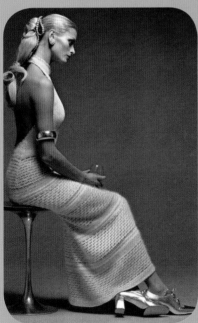

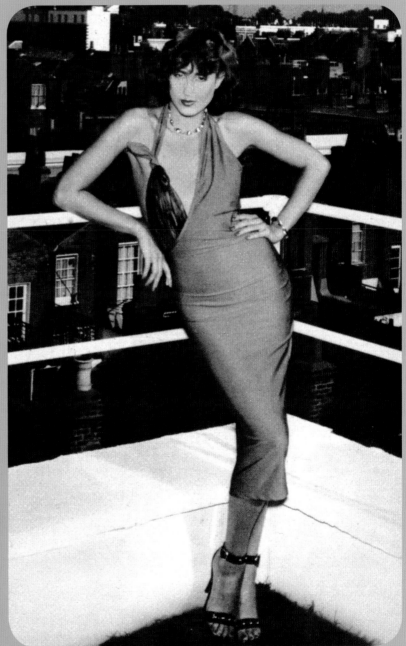

Silk

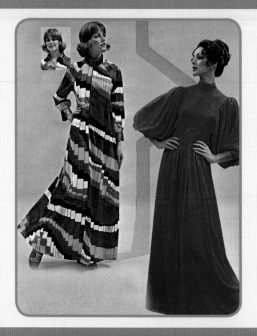

From elegant, body-hugging jersey dresses and jumpsuits to free-flowing evening gowns and kaftans, silk became one of the most popular fabrics in fashion throughout the decade.

Tuxedo Suit

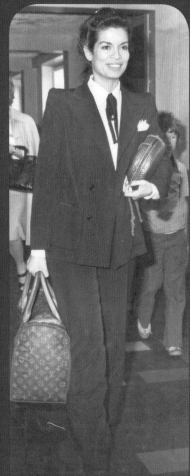

Those seeking a more understated but elegant evening look went for the tuxedo suit. Yves Saint Laurent launched his famous female tuxedo suit, Le Smoking, in 1966, which was an instant success and the precursor for the modern-day trouser suit. But it was Mick Jagger's wife, Bianca, who became famed for wearing versions of the androgynous attire throughout the seventies, setting the style bar high with her striking looks and effortless chic.

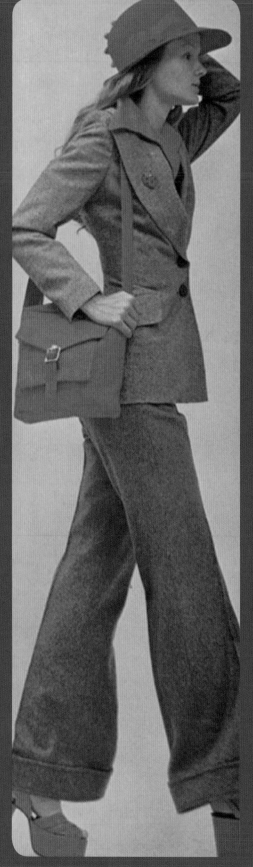

Tattoo Fashion

Issey Miyake's 1971 collection of body tights were a glimpse of what was to come with body-con fashion in the following years. Skin tight, the one piece represented a second skin and was decorated with various designs including tattoos of cult singer/musicians Janis Joplin and Jimi Hendrix.

Pan's People

All-girl dance troupe Pan's People were a regular feature on the BBC programme *Top of The Pops*. Their interpretive dance routines were performed in elaborate costumes, which inspired many young women's fashion tastes on the dance floors of nightclubs and discos in the UK.

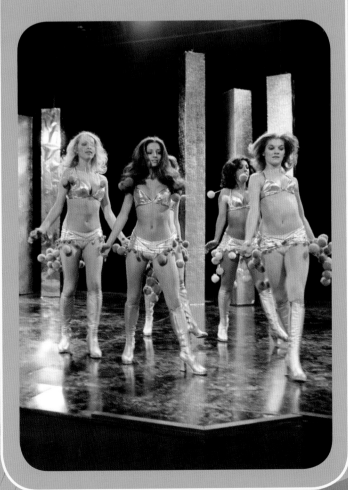

From Office to Dance Floor....

The concept of wearing fashionable separates meant both sexes could adapt their look for an easy transition from day to evening wear. Independent ladies could move from the workplace to dinner and then on to the disco in the same outfit, with only the smallest of tweaks to their accessories. One such garment that allowed this freedom was the iconic wrap dress designed by Diane Von Furstenberg in 1972. The overwhelming success of this design and its subsequent influence on women's fashion saw Furstenberg declared the most remarkable woman since Coco Chanel in an article about her in *Newsweek* Magazine in 1976. She replaced Gerald Ford on the front cover, even though he had just won his first Republican presidential primary.

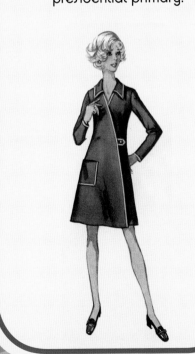

1970s MEN'S EVENING WEAR

Designers of men's evening wear looked to the past for inspiration. They produced a wide range of styles: Victorian dress shirts, elements of Edwardian romance and Teddy Boy chic were revived with velvet trim, embroidery and ruffles. The single-breasted suit was shunned in favour of the double, and waistcoats again became important, with the shield shape (bottom right) fashionable later in the decade. Straight-end bow ties were worn with the vintage favourite wing collar, which was now a soft attachment and more comfortable to wear. This was finished with shiny patent lace ups. As the 1980s loomed, the tuxedo took on a simpler, sleeker cut, losing the fancy excesses and adopting a more contemporary feel.

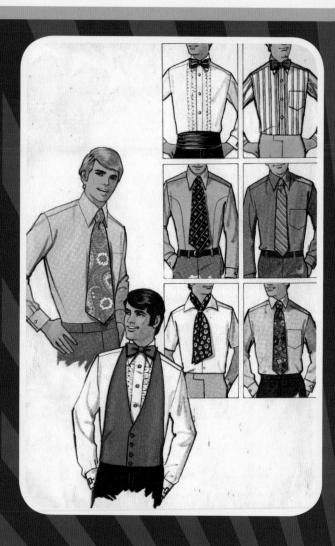

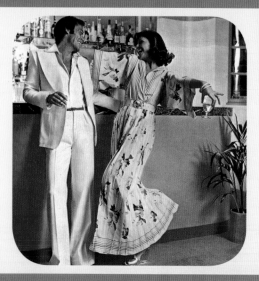

Saturday Night Fever

Donning your disco pants was obligatory on a Saturday night and they had to form part of a smart but not overly formal three-piece suit. The cut of men's evening wear had fallen more in line with that of a leisure suit – adjusted for a more body-hugging silhouette and much less formal than a tuxedo. Chests were bared with shirts left unbuttoned and trousers left little to the imagination, only becoming loose and flared from the knee down.

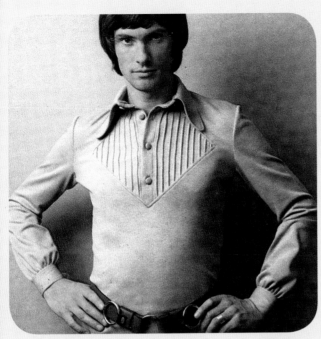

Glam Rock

Much of th public had strict ideas about what constituted traditonal dress for men and women. Glam rock challenged this as men started to wear clothes and colours more commonly seen on women. It was Marc Bolan (below) who made a glamorous glitter-and-sequin clad entrance to the stage of *Top of The Pops*, setting a fashion precedent that saw men reaching for satin trousers, hair dye and make-up.

Collared!

The seventies embraced the classic straight shirt collar, which became wider and longer than ever before. The early part of the decade saw collars with an average 7 cm (2¾ in) point length – the distance from the collar points to the collar band – but this increased dramatically for dress shirts which were worn unbuttoned into a deep V.

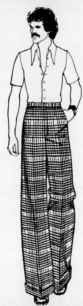

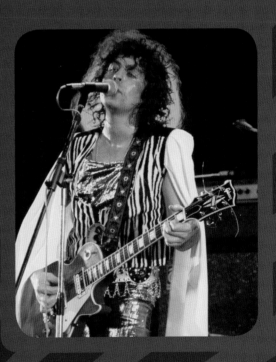

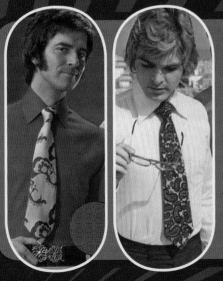

Done Up Like a Kipper

Men's necks were adorned with a variety of styles but it is the kipper tie that is most closely associated with the seventies. Worn as part of both day and evening wear, the breadth of the kipper tie was enormous, even trumping the widths seen on zoot-suit wearers in the forties. Michael Fish (not the weatherman!) of the shop Mr Fish in London's Carnaby Street – famously noted for his outlandish designs – was the one responsible for their creation.

1970s SHOES

The stiletto shape was banished to shoe heaven in the seventies and became virtually non-existent in new collections. Fashion still reached towering heights, with the arrival of platform shoes and boots adding several inches to the height of both men and women. The designs were not entirely new, but it was in the seventies that platform designs really escalated to universal popularity. Another favourite style worn by both men and women was the clog. Traditionally made of wood and worn as heavy work shoes, the clogs of the 1970s had stacked soles and heels and were made from a variety of materials.

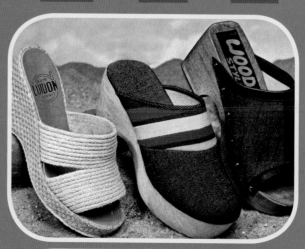

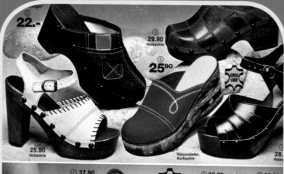

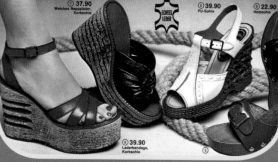

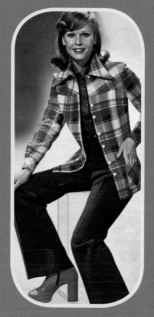

New Heights

Platforms were just that, a platform on which the wearer would be elevated, with the block sole and heel sometimes highlighted in multicoloured stripes. The bravery of the wearer would dictate the elevation levels, which could be anything from 5 to 7.5 cm (2-3 in) right up to 9 cm (nearly 4 in). Stiletto variations existed where the sole alone would be stacked and accompanied by a pencil-thin towering heel, a look that went on to become intrinsically associated with the sex industry. But it was the wooden sandal platform with simple leather buckled straps that was most widely worn.

High Heels, Sir?

During a decade when fashion was becoming increasingly androgynous, it wasn't long before men's shoes diversified from being either flat or platform and started to become available with varying heel heights, similar to that of a lady's block heel court shoe. The trend was embraced by the young and fashionable as well as by those who were vertically challenged. But the style attracted a great deal of criticism from the more traditionally minded, who considered the shoes one step too far for their masculinity!

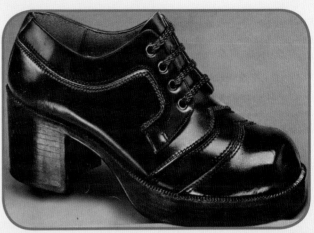

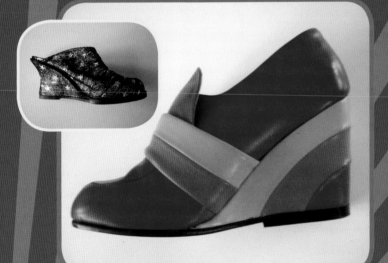

Sandals

The sandal is one of the oldest designs of shoe, with known examples dating back 10,000 years. The open toe and sometimes backless design not only complemented the comfort-loving hippie trends of the day but also allowed the shoe to be thoroughly unisex, catapulting it into virtually everyone's wardrobe regardless of age or sex. Sandals exposed many uncared-for toes and heels, which could look unsightly. More often than not, individuals reached for the pumice stone but many simply reached for socks. The sock and sandal combo is probably one of the most ridiculed looks in fashion history – but some seem to just love it!

Wedges

Like platforms, wedge shoes have a long history in fashion in both ancient times and in the 1930s, when Salvatore Ferragamo brought the design to the Italians. The wedge was an alternative to the platform, usually for ladies looking for a comfortable fusion of height and practicality. The shape of the shoe positioned the wearer's balance on to the ball of the foot and offered stability when walking.

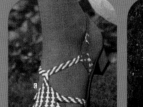

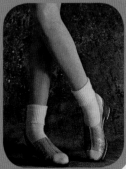

1970s SPORTSWEAR

There was a great diversity in leisurewear by the seventies, with specialist 'sportwear' brands establishing themselves alongside the fashion aristocracy. Many sports companies evolved to become must-have brands as more and more sportswear was worn as informal fashion ensembles. Americans led the way with casual apparel, with designers such as Geoffrey Beene and Bill Blass bringing sportswear styling into everyday clothing design. Ralph Lauren and Perry Ellis were creating fashion tsunamis stateside, not to mention Vera Maxwell, and Anne Klein, who was employing Donna Karan as her associate designer in 1971.

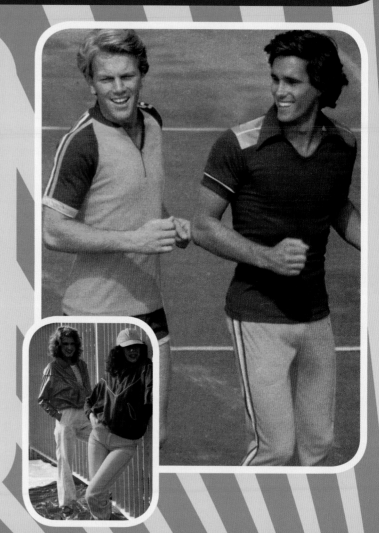

Athlete's Feet

The trainer or sneaker evolved from being the specialist footwear of athletes into something more fashion oriented. Brands fought for market domination, vying to sponsor sports celebrities who would increase their following. Adidas and Puma famously agreed to make Brazilian footballer Pelè 'off limits' for the 1970 World Cup, but Puma secretly reneged and when Pelè halted match proceedings to tie his shoe laces, the world was fixed on the Puma logo, sending sales rocketing!

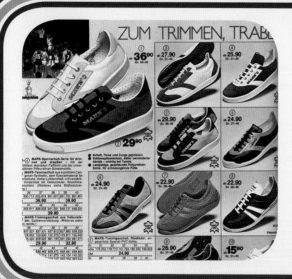

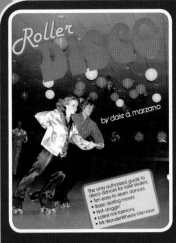
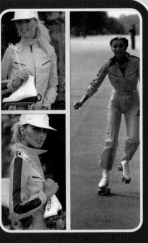
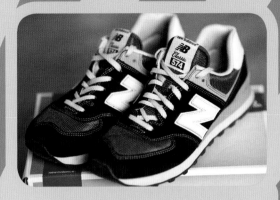

Roll On By

Traditional sports like tennis, cricket and golf remained popular, but alternative activities were also gaining growing audiences. Technological advances in plastics meant roller-skate design could give the wearer more control over their movements and roller skating soon became part of the music sensation of the decade – disco. Arenas were built solely for roller discos and people flocked to the dance floor. Women wore leotards and cut-off jeans with bright socks. Spandex and shorts weren't just the reserve of women though as men donned skin-tight T-shirts and satin shorts with white piping!

Balancing Act

New Balance was a Boston-based sports footwear company established at the turn of the century. At the start of the 1970s the company was struggling to maintain its business despite the thriving sportswear market.
But, by sheer luck, Boston became the hub of running in America – giving the company a much-needed boost and making its footwear a fashion favourite.

Need for Speed

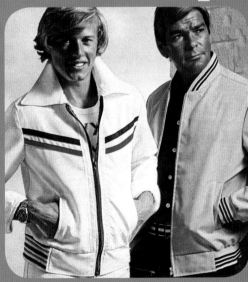
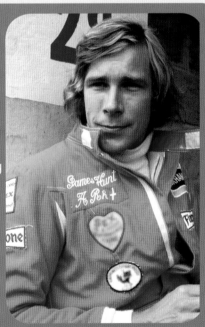

Many different varieties of racing gripped the nation in the seventies. Sport's figures such as Eddy Merckx and James Hunt (right) dominated cycling and motor racing respectively, and what they wore both on and off the race tracks became woven into the fashions of the day.

1970s ACCESSORIES

For diverse subcultures and street fashions, a little accessorizing made a big statement. Both costume and fine jewellery had a heavy ethnic feel that merged elements of nature into its shapes and colours. Enamelling was extremely popular, which supported the artisan vibe storming the fashion world. Hats were back and, with the decade's penchant for basking in the sun, the design of your sunglasses was as important as the rest of your outfit.

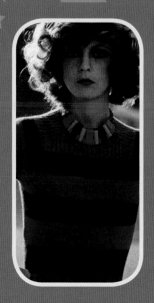

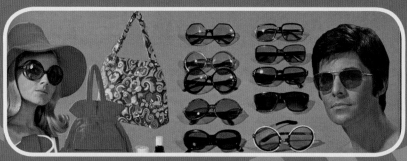

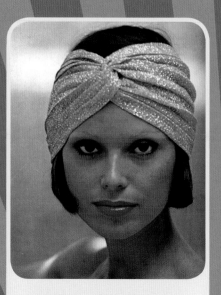

Turbans

Whether you wound a scarf around your head or donned a more traditional pull-on pleated version, the turban was very much in vogue in the seventies. An extension of the ethnic fashions being seen everywhere, the turban was an easy-to- wear accessory for both day and evening wear.

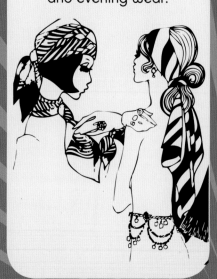

Badgered!

Wearing a badge had long been an expression of achievement or an affiliation to a group. But in the seventies anti-establishment figures catapulted the badge into fashion. Widely seized upon by hippies, punks also used badges to demonstrate their disdain for conformity.

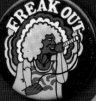

Get the Look with Hannah

Much of 1970s fashion has stood the test of time, and the decade is one of the most revisited by contemporary designers. Original seventies Dior sunglasses are highly collectable and will be a key piece in your vintage wardrobe, guaranteed to get lots of wear.

Bags of Fun

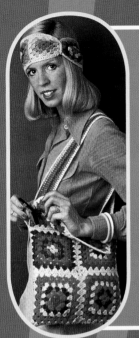
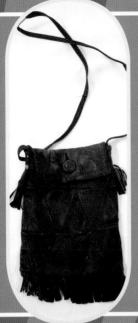

Everyday bags were becoming more utilitarian with shoulder bags being the most popular style for the working woman, based on functionality and ease of wearing. Oversizing extended from clothes to bags, with simple shapes and two-piece tapestry bags the nod to the passion for artisan design seen abroad. Cartier launched its luxury Leather Collection in 1974, choosing a rich shade of burgundy that appealed to those seeking exclusive branding on their arm. More affordable names followed, offering ranges in alternative natural materials. Hessian and straw were 'in' and, as with most other aspects of fashion, ethnic patterns and shapes provided influence.

Jewel in the Crown

Jewellery was a popular accessory, with a trend for layering pieces. Hippies favoured wood, stones and crystals as well as recycled head bands, which were often customized with artificial flowers or broken jewellery. The more 'all-American girl' would opt for gold or silver, while punks embraced the less conventional choosing kilt pins as brooches and wearing clothing studs and safety pins as earrings.

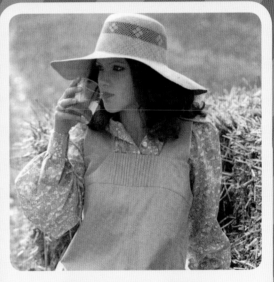

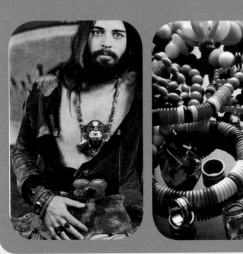

Turn Up the Heat

The summer of 1976 was the hottest on record in the UK. This unprecedented heatwave injected new life into the millinery industry, which had suffered a serious downturn in the sixties. As temperatures soared the demand increased for both practical, cool and stylish head wear propelling the summer hat to the fashion echelons. The floppy, wide-brimmed hat became synonymous with the decade and was soon adapted for all seasons.

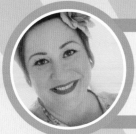

1970s GET THE LOOK WITH HANNAH

Whether you prefer disco to punk or glam rock to fresh-faced Boho Chic, the *seventies* gave you the freedom to experiment and was finally starting to incorporate black hair and make-up styling into the mainstream. Beauty in this period features the fresh-faced 'barely there' look. The trend was all about accentuation rather than emphasis, which is much harder to achieve than applying a full-on night-time look. However, with the right tools it can be done. The decade also saw trends which harked back to the past, with make-up styles originally seen on 1920s flapper girls and 1940s Hollywood sirens.

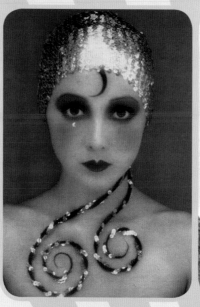

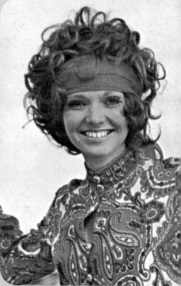

Eyes of an Angel

The characters in *Charlie's Angels* were the epitome of seventies chic with their tousled hair and sun-kissed skin. To achieve that look use a gradual tan moisturizer to develop a natural healthy glow. Eye shadow should be light brown shades for fairer skin, and a matte gold on darker skin. Darker browns can be added to the outer corners of the eye. Natural brows have a gentle arch and are typically quite thick, so keep them groomed and, if necessary, use a brow powder to fill any gaps. Use black or brown mascara to separate top and bottom lashes. For luminescence, use a highlighter that will help catch the light. This should be applied only on areas that you want to enhance (under brows, outer edge of cheek bones, top lip). Use the highlighter across the collar bone to emphasize your shoulders and décolletage.

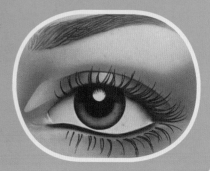

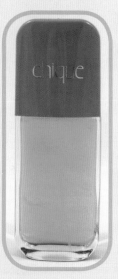

Heaven Scent

Women wore sweet and floral fragrances with perfumes like *Miss Worth* (House of Worth), *Eau De Patou* (Jean Patou) and *Babe* (Fabergé). Men opted for light citrus notes such as *Polo* (Ralph Lauren) and *Monsieur Rochas* (Rochas) or continued to splash on classic *Brut*.

Heavenly Hair

To complement the 'barely there' look, hair should look natural and gently tousled. Rough dry clean hair with a hairdryer. Using a salt spray, lightly spritz your entire head. Divide hair into rough sections and plait. On a medium to low setting, use a hairdryer to dry the salt spray into the hair. Undo the plaits and run your fingers (not a brush or comb) through the curls to separate them. Use straightening irons to flatten any bendy curls. Finally, rub a pea size amount of matte paste or serum into the ends of your hair for that classic 'bed hair' look.

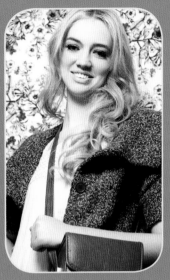
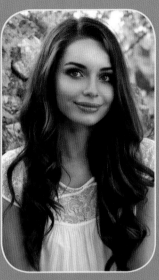

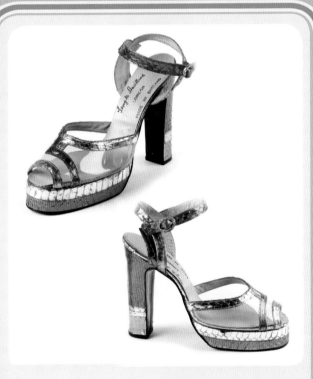

Chic Feet

Look out for greatly prized Terry de Havilland (above) and Manolo Blahnik shoes. Both designers were big names at this time with de Havilland famed for his platforms and wedges and Blahnik for his evening-wear sandals often in metallic shades.

Plain Rude

For the iconic rude boy look, be brave and take your hair clippers down to a No.1 setting and cut your hair all over. Team your new look with a checked shirt, braces, drain-pipe jeans and Dr Marten shin-high boots, topped off with a Harrington jacket and you're ready to ska the night away!

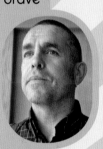

Fringe Benefits

For a more 'seventies' fringe, make sure it starts quite far back (at the centre-top of your head) and is blow dried under to finish beneath your eyebrows. Don't limit a fringe just to your hairstyle – customizing your clothes by adding fringing will give them an authentic period twist!

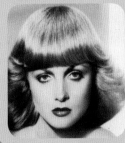

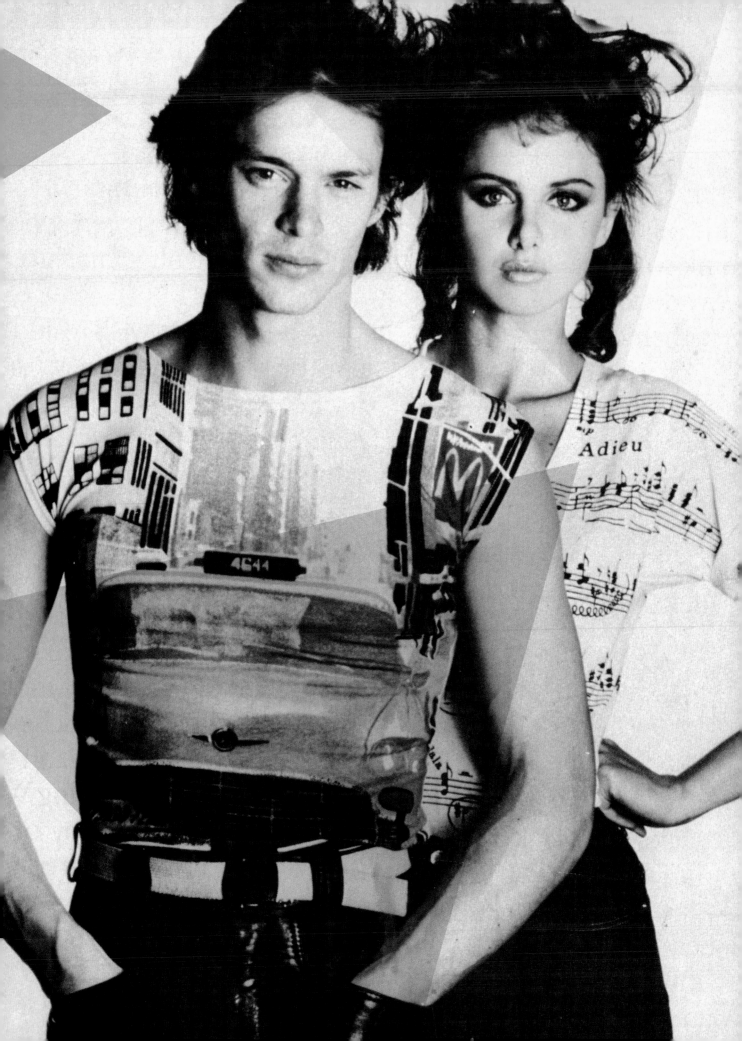

1980s

As a decade obsessed with status, the eighties brought excess into all areas of fashion. From the strength of your fragrance to the width of your shoulder pads, more was simply a must. The theatrics of fashion created factions of image-conscious individuals, competing to make the most striking statement on the street and in the neon-lit nightclubs. Their medley of alternative dress was a visual treasure chest from which you could become a real fashion magpie.

With so much focus concentrated on the cut of your clothes, it was inevitable that the cult of the 'body beautiful' would come to the fore, bringing with it a mania for fitness. In the US Jane Fonda made eyes pop with her 'workout', while Britain's offering was its daily breakfast aerobic sessions with 'Mad Lizzie' — everyone reached for the Spandex and Lycra and a new wave of 'fitness fashion' began.

Although music had always been connected with fashion, it was the launch of a radical new television station in 1981 that cemented the fusion. MTV was the first channel of its kind, dedicated to playing music videos which were to become an exciting platform for the latest clothes. The highly stylized looks seen in these new video accompaniments to chart hits helped high-street sales rocket as young and old went in search of must-have image-defining outfits. The concept of what it was to be 'fashionable' had seemingly changed for ever by the 1980s, with a lack of conformity seen as cutting edge and therefore bestowing kudos.

1987 saw fundamental economic disruption create a temporary tightening of shopper's purse strings, which impacted fashion-house production. But by the end of the decade the UK was experiencing a financial boom once again. The people were waiting for the imminent demise of a long-standing and increasingly hated government, and under the grip of a newly established 'rave scene', which was to reshape fashion once more for the nineties.

1980s WOMEN'S DAY WEAR

An increasingly powerful female workforce in the eighties created a demand for fashion that was both up to date, functional and smart enough to serve the new wave of female executives striding in to formerly all-male environments, from the boardroom to Downing Street. Fashion day wear had become so broad in its interpretation that, aided by the sheer volume of mix and match separates, women were developing a real uniqueness in their everyday appearance as never before.

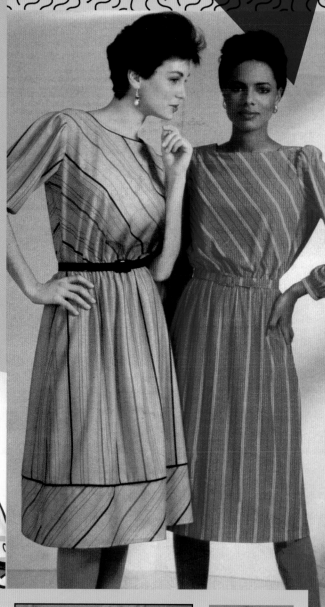

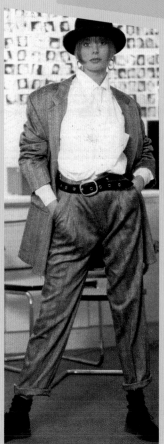

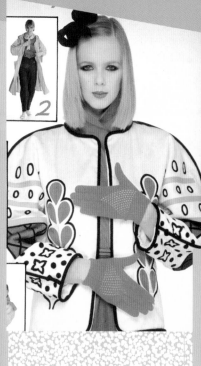

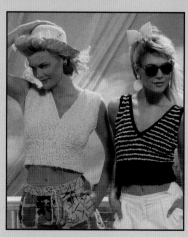

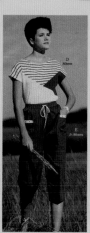

DENIM DELIGHTS

Historically a heavy-duty work wear material, denim had evolved to be something of a staple in everyone's wardrobe by the 1980s. The passion for the fabric had by this time extended into its use to construct jackets, shirts, dresses, skirts, waistcoats and, of course, a variety of jean cuts and styles. Levi and Wrangler used the importance of your body shape to market their different denim wears, bringing much attention to the derrière, and in a very short space of time denim became 'designer'. The prevailing style in the eighties favoured a loose fit towards the top half of the jeans with a tapered leg which would be tightly and very neatly rolled above the ankle. All over the world, fashion houses were picking up on the popularity of denim and creating collections which were immediately embraced for their practicality and brand-name kudos. With the trend for overtly

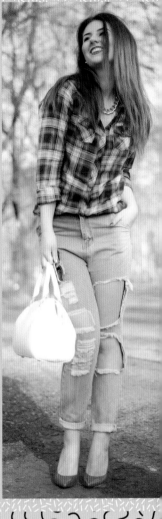

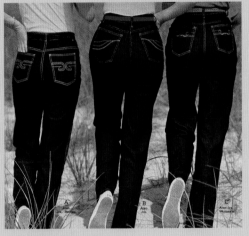

displaying where your clothes were from, the brand patch typically found on the rear right of jeans was usually colourful and detailed. The continued popularity of denim resulted in all sorts of experiments with the fabric and gave us bleached, stonewash, heavily pigmented, and differing shades of blue. Also on offer were varying leg widths, and detailed ripping and fading to emulate a 'worn in' look. It is no wonder then that the trend for 'double denim' (wearing multiple garments made from the fabric) became synonymous with the decade.

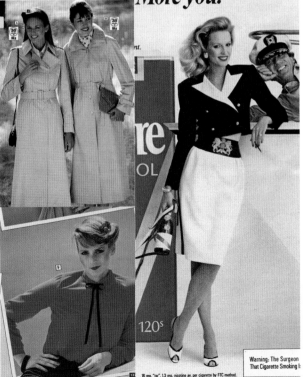

THE POWER SUIT

The concept of the 'business woman' was evolving, and this new breed demanded a wardrobe that was as serious as their determination to succeed. There were several popular shapes and cuts, which were influenced by the revered designers of yesteryear. The cropped box jacket finished high at the natural waist, and was paired with fitted skirts that finished just above the knee. Blouses or shirts were worn tucked in to accentuate the waist and came in a variety of colours and patterns, with thick shoulder pads to create width across the shoulders. Alternative shaping leaned more towards men's suits, in particular those from the twenties and forties, with long jackets, notch lapels and waistcoats. Trousers with high waists had wide legs and front pleats with wide turn-up hems. The trick to retaining an air of femininity was down to the colours and materials used. Suits were made in delicate fabrics and light neutral shades, giving a much softer edge.

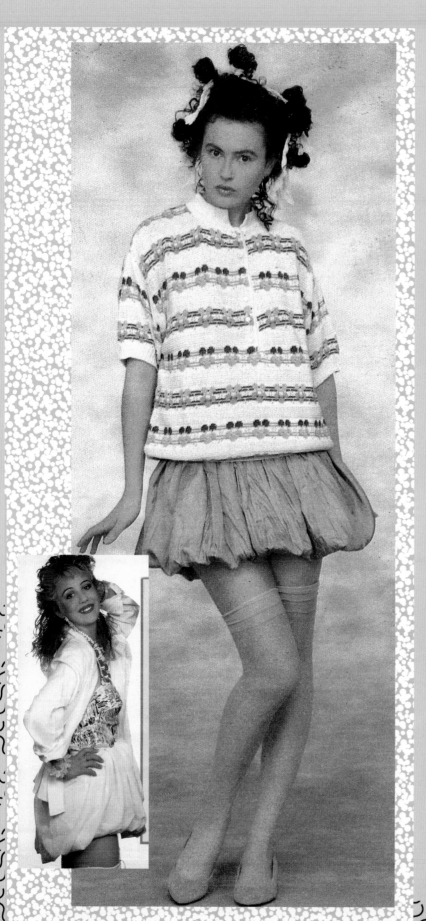

I'LL HUFF AND I'LL PUFF

Mini skirts had been evolving ever since they made their debut in the sixties, and towards the end of the eighties the 'puffball' made its debut. Credited to French designer Christian Lacroix, the puffball skirt was essentially a medium length of fabric that was doubled over, slightly gathered and finished with a plain waistband, creating a puffball mushroom shape (hence the name). Although its origins lay in haute couture, the style was swiftly adopted by mainstream clothing manufacturers as a 'young' trend and worn with jumpers and blouses as casual day wear. The popularity of the skirt meant it wasn't long before it was being sported by pop stars like the UK's Bananarama, and the trend extended to outfits seen on the disco dance floor. Don't confuse the puffball with the rah-rah skirt which was also worn a lot in the eighties. The rah-rah was a layered fabric skirt that owed its origins to the short skirts worn by cheerleaders.

BIG & BOLD & BRIGHT

The 'big look' of the seventies had carried over into the eighties, with oversize chunky knitwear designs becoming ever more outlandish. Vivienne Westwood had showcased a variety of knitted garments with deliberate repeated holes in them and an asymmetric, twisted construction that pushed boundaries and created a new take on how to wear wool. This was picked up and developed by other designers and knitting-pattern producers, who used vivid colours and multiple stitch patterns.

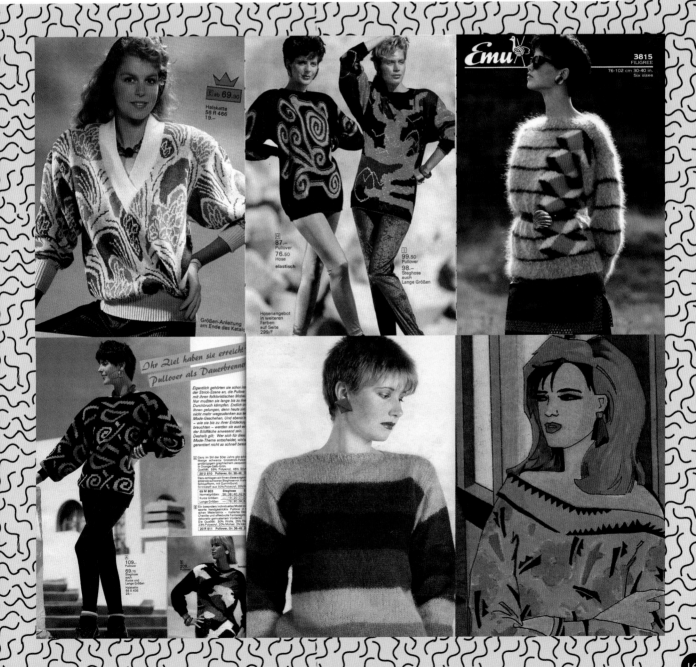

Generally, fashion in the 1980s could be seen to veer towards conventionality. Power-dressing, Yuppies (young, upwardly-mobile professionals) and shoulder pads held sway in the mainstream. The flip side of this was the ultimate word in informality: on the street the often purposefully shapeless logo and message T-shirt prevailed. Some designers, such as Katherine Hamnett, sought to inspire protest, with examples such as '58% Don't want Pershing', while flavour-of-the-moment pop stars such as Frankie Goes to Hollywood expanded their brand through printed statements emblazoned proudly across the chests of the world's teenagers, from Copenhagen to Bangalore.

1980s T-SHIRTS

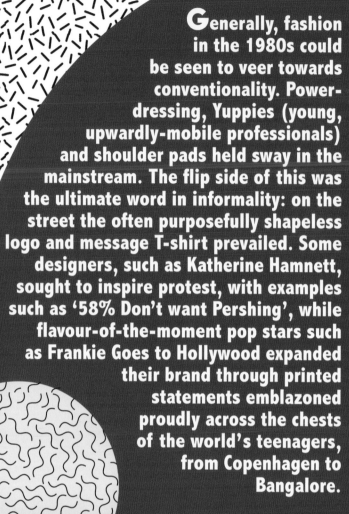

In this, the decade of the clothes-catalogue shopper, the primary-coloured, abstract designs that sold off the page cruised the streets, the beaches and the clubs. Worn baggy and well below the waist, the eighties T-shirt shouted loudly that it intended to stay for the whole decade.

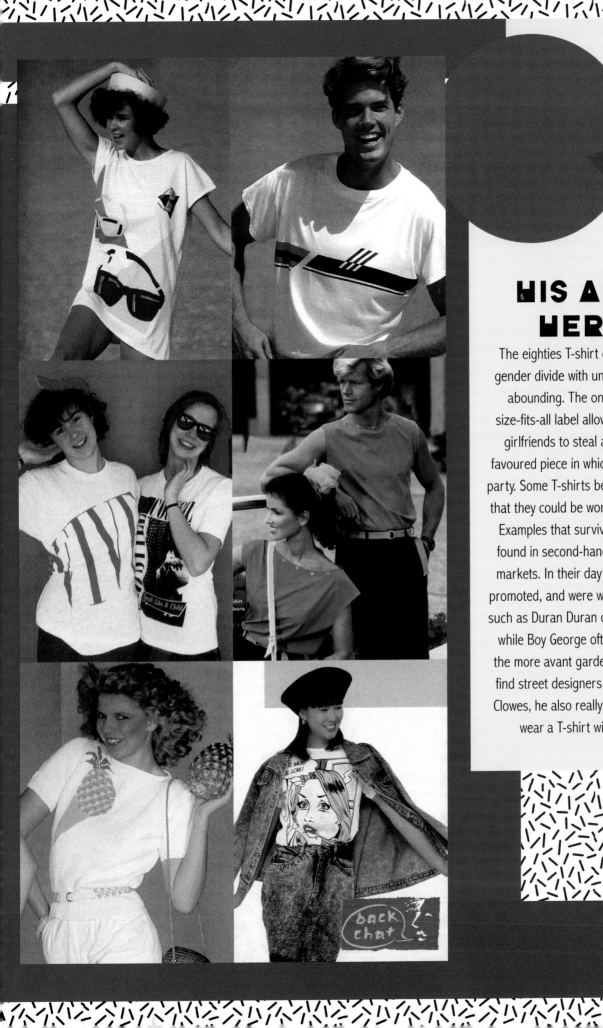

HIS AND HERS

The eighties T-shirt crossed the gender divide with unisex designs abounding. The one-(large)-size-fits-all label allowed a million girlfriends to steal a partner's favoured piece in which to sleep or party. Some T-shirts became so long that they could be worn as a dress. Examples that survive are easily found in second-hand shops and markets. In their day these shirts promoted, and were worn by, bands such as Duran Duran or Wham!, and while Boy George often favoured the more avant garde and hard to find street designers such as Sue Clowes, he also really knew how to wear a T-shirt with style.

1980s MEN'S DAY WEAR

Much like their female counterparts, gents were just as concerned with their image throughout the eighties with colourful jumpers, slim fit trousers and polo shirts among the most popular day wear seen during the decade. Elite-end fashion was tacked onto the pendulum of sexual equality that was bringing women into the high-earning, male-dominated environments. Staff-room coffee tables were covered in copies of *i-D* and *Paper* magazines alongside *GQ* and *Vogue*, with multi-million pound advertising and celebrity endorsement influencing fashion choices more than ever before.

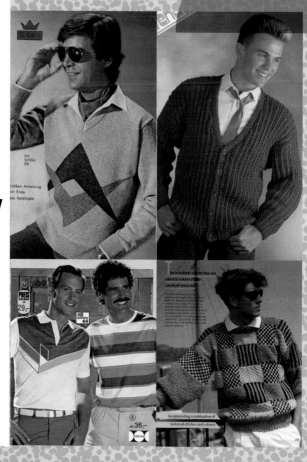

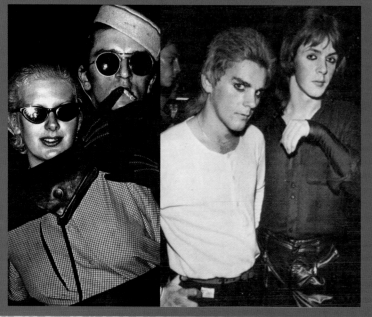

HARD TIMES

Adopted into mainstream fashion terminology 'buffalo' is Caribbean slang for 'rude boy' and references the essence behind the fashion label of the late Ray Petri. The designer created a sylish but functional street style and the 'hard look' acted as a catalyst for 'contemporary' styling that is abundant in independent fashion magazines today. The fine line between feminine and masculine detailing was a point of constant experimentation for Petri, chiming perfectly with eighties' liberal style sensitivities at a time when fashion boundaries were being stretched.

HARD TIMES

HOMME FROM HOME

Rei Kawakubo had been established in the field of fashion for several years before she expanded into menswear, launching her very first line of Comme Des Garçonne Homme in 1978. Lampooned as 'wacky', the eighties designs saw models on the catwalk wearing oversized, mainly black creations that were deemed monastic or dubbed 'Hiroshima chic'. The cut of Japanese fashion, which stirred interest from around the globe, ignored mainstream tailoring, instead leaning towards a more deconstructed approach like that of established and revered Western designer Vivienne Westwood. The designs diverged from many of the earlier collections that were aimed at mainstream audiences, but that only added to the label's exclusivity and alternative styling gradually took off in the eighties. European designers started referencing foreign cultural dress in their pattern cutting and using vivid splashes of colour to create a mark of difference in their collections, which were showcased alongside power suits and huge shoulder pads on the fashion stages.

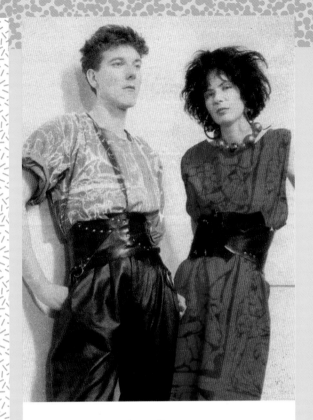

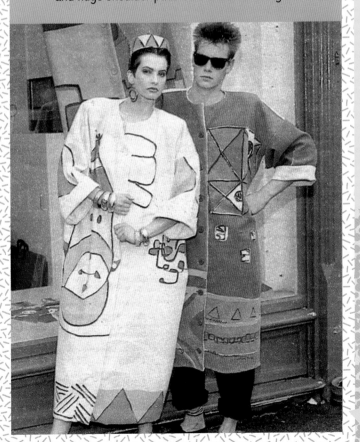

GETTING LEATHERED

Leather was used extensively to create unisex clothing throughout the decade, from patches on knitwear to trousers and jackets. The 'MJ' jacket is a classic take on the leather jacket worn by Michael Jackson in the 'Thriller' music video, which propelled the style to the forefront of fashion must haves for men and boys alike.

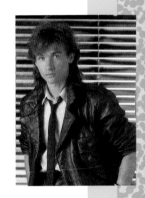

GET THE LOOK WITH HANNAH

If leather is looked after it can last a lifetime, however in extreme environments like damp or heat the protein bonds that make the material can crack. Always check vintage leather to see if it is brittle. If it is, there is every chance it will tear with no chance of repair. Use a good leather oil to keep garments supple.

MIAMI NICE

Television and advertising became more and more influential in the eighties, marked by the launch of Channel 4 in the UK in 1982, and Sky at the end of the decade in 1989. The expansion brought with it a wealth of programmes with characters that gripped audiences and served to dictate their wardrobe choices. None did more so than characters Sonny Crockett and Ricardo Tubbs from *Miami Vice,* who were to become male style icons for the decade. Their fashion sense both on and off screen became synonymous with the linen trousers, T-shirt and lightweight sports jacket their characters regularly wore. Gianni Versace, Hugo Boss and Vittorio Ricci were just some of the big names consulted by costume designers for the show to ensure that the outfits had a European feel, and the deliberate use of pastel colours complemented the show's Art Deco backdrop of Miami. The programme spawned several collections for the general public, including the company Take Six, which created a line of Miami Vice dinner jackets, and US store Macy's, which opened a Miami Vice section in its young men's department. As a result, millions of men from around the world bought brushed cotton suits in pastel shades and rolled up their sleeves in homage to the crime-busting duo.

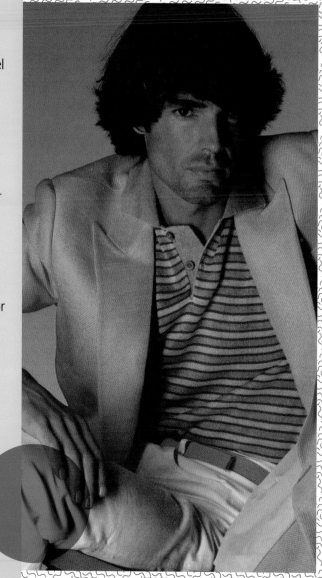

ALL RAPPED UP

Multiple subcultures existed throughout the eighties, each with a unique sense of style defining its affiliation to a particular fashion and music choice. Stateside gave us Hip Hop in the late seventies, which bloomed in the eighties and expanded across the pond to shape British fashion ideas. Men wore dark trousers, jeans or tracksuit bottoms with hooded tracksuit jackets or leather jackets, accessorized with baseball caps, fedora hats and chunky gold chains.

YOU CAN DO IT!
BREAKDANCE

AS ADVERTISED ON T...

...WALK, BODYPOP AND ELECTRIC BOOGIE

FEATURES
THE NEW YORK CITY
BREAKERS
ALEX & THE CITY CREW

HIP HOP BODYPOP TO BREAKDANCE PARTY, AUTOMATIC, ROCKIT, LETS HEAR IT FOR THE BOY, SPECIAL BREAKMIX.

(K-tel)

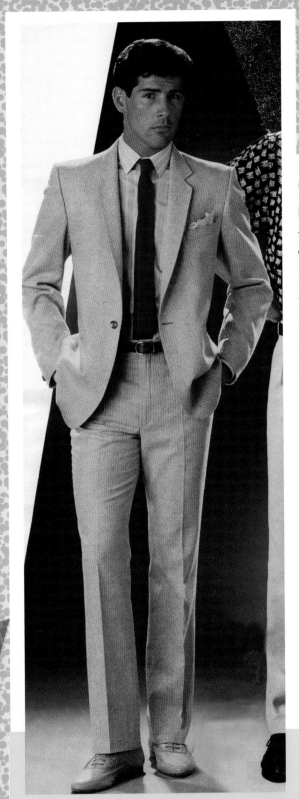

CITY SLICKERS

High-flying men felt they needed statement suits which shouted the wearer's competency and confidence in all things business. While the traditional colour palette was still in existence, it became commonplace during the eighties for business wear to come in a wide range of lighter shades. The cut of many contemporary designer suits represented the trend for body awareness, with classic-cut single-breasted jackets with wide sloping shoulders. This accentuated, or at least suggested, a manly triangular upper body shape. Trousers were slim fitting (although not as snug as in the previous decade), and it was perfectly acceptable for trouser hems to be rolled up, exposing sockless ankles.

BRAND MAGIC

The eighties saw a surge in established high-street fashion brand names being emblazoned all over their garments. The opportunity to wear something from a top brand, and let the world know exactly where it came from, made some trends more about who the garment was by than its actual cut and design. This was particularly true of Benetton and Gap; their casual wear T-shirts and sweatshirts carried the brand name right across the chest, making the wearer an inadvertent billboard and promoting sales even further.

GET THE LOOK WITH HANNAH

A pastel-coloured, long-sleeved jumper tied loosely around your shoulders will give you that instant eighties preppie look, especially if it is teamed with a vivid polo shirt and beige chinos.

1980s WOMEN'S EVENING WEAR

The quest for fashion individuality had grown enormously by the eighties creating a vast number of designers vying to make their mark. Popular designers such as Thierry Mugler focused on structural composition, earning him much positive acclaim, alongside Christian Lacroix who became the yougest couturier in the business in 1986. The competition was fierce, with the evening-wear label becoming just as important as the actual design. There was an air of theatre that drew reference from the past, challenging mainstream design and creating a more avant-garde approach. However, it was the cocktail dress that was set to make a comeback.

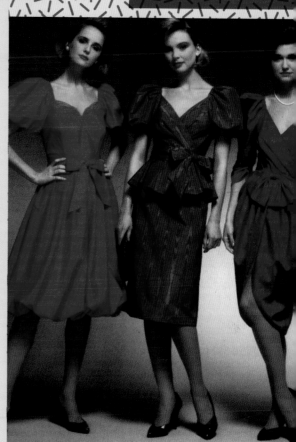

THE PEOPLE'S PRINCESS

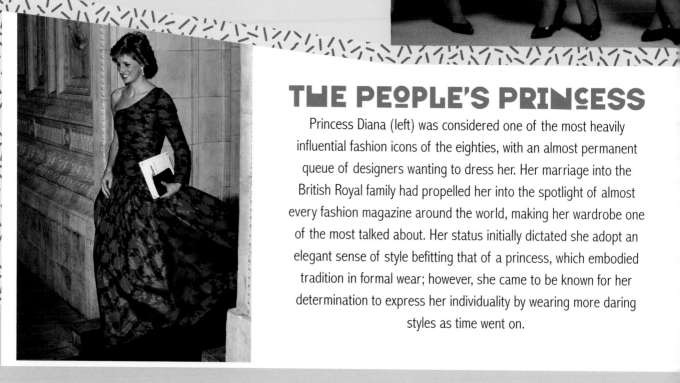

Princess Diana (left) was considered one of the most heavily influential fashion icons of the eighties, with an almost permanent queue of designers wanting to dress her. Her marriage into the British Royal family had propelled her into the spotlight of almost every fashion magazine around the world, making her wardrobe one of the most talked about. Her status initially dictated she adopt an elegant sense of style befitting that of a princess, which embodied tradition in formal wear; however, she came to be known for her determination to express her individuality by wearing more daring styles as time went on.

ALL THAT GLITTERS

Alexis Colby strutted onto our screens in the eighties and brought with her one of the most revered wardrobes of the decade. Played by actress Joan Collins, the *Dynasty* character played a scorned woman with a vindictive streak and a passion for looking fabulous at all times. The character's costume was always figure-flattering, featuring evening gowns influenced by forties and fifties design. The sweetheart neckline and nipped-in waists seen on vintage 'wiggle dresses' was incorporated, with enormous shoulder pads, and given a modern twist with copious scatterings of sparkle in the form of diamantès, gold chain edging or more commonly, thousands of sequins — a look repeatedly emulated by would-be divas and glamour-seekers throughout the decade.

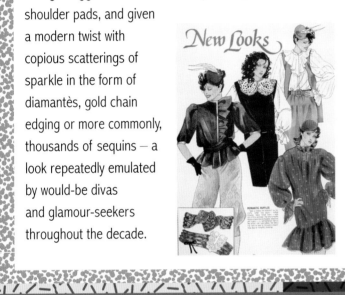

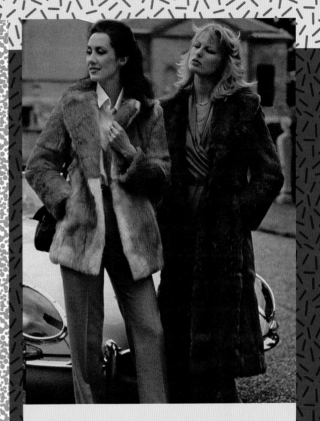

REAL OR FAKE?

With women's fashion looking to appeal to the new wave of empowered females, the eighties embraced bold animal prints and furs like never before. In particular, the brown and yellow tones of leopard markings led the way in the fashion jungle. This did, however, bring controversy as animal rights organization PETA campaigned to abolish the slaughter of animals for their pelts; the fashion industry responded with the speedy development and production of realistic fake fur.

CUTTING EDGE

The cut of women's clothing in the eighties seemed to echo the fight for equality with men, too. The typical 'alpha male' physique — an upside-down triangle — was widely replicated, with large shoulder pads and raglan sleeves in all aspects of women's fashion.

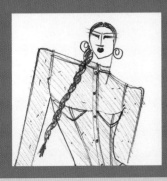

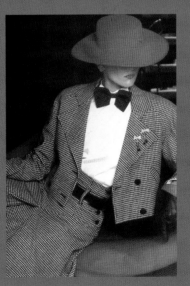

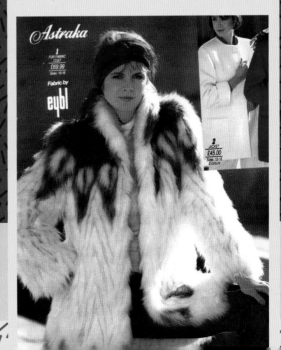

1980s MEN'S EVENING WEAR

Men's evening wear had all but moved away from the traditional in terms of what was considered fashionable in the 1980s. There was still a demand for strict formality in certain circles and for this, the tuxedo shape would once again change to fit the times. However, most designers were taking a much more progressive approach. The boundaries of men's evening wear had been shifting since the sixties. Now, with the notion that fashion did not have to be dictated by popular consensus, materials, colour and design became more experimental, incorporating influences from contemporary art and music to create a theatrical quality.

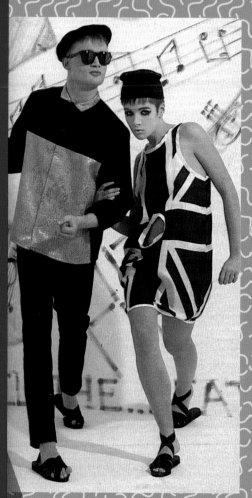

RAVE NATION

Rave music had taken the fashion industry by storm in the late eighties, with the 'smiley face' becoming the official logo of the scene. The popularity of 'acid house' meant men's informal evening wear adopted a look previously only associated with leisure pursuits or the gym. It was around this time that fashion group Red or Dead first came to the fore, with rave culture and dance music a heavy influence on early designs.

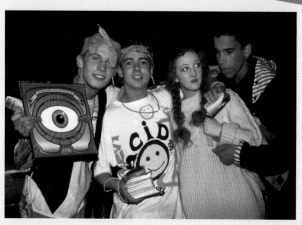

A FINE ROMANCE

The deliberate androgyny of New Wave and New Romantic fashion was intrinsically linked to popular music, with roots in The Blitz club in London during 1979 and 1980. The club itself was positioned not far from the fashion HQ that is Central Saint Martins and therefore attracted a creative clientele of students and graduates like Stephen Linard, who turned the club into a fashion catwalk as much as a place to dance. It wasn't long before some of the leading designers of the time began using the club to showcase their work, which served to ramp up the competition for creativity. Sue Clowes was famously approached to design for Boy George, who along with the likes of Billy Idol and Spandau Ballet were regulars at the club. Stevie Stewart and David Holah who founded Bodymap, Lee Bowery, Judi Frankland, Dinny Hall and Kim Bowen were among a small group of fashion creatives who dominated the party scene in the eighties and are considered some of the most influential individuals of fashion, not just then but of all time. Inspiration was sought from absolutely everywhere and included controversial ecclesiastical garb, such as habits and dog collars, which inevitably provoked a reaction. Borrowing elements from punk and Edwardian flamboyance, New Romantic fashion was a mish-mash of satin, silk, lace, frills and other gathered materials which incorporated oversizing with soft colour palettes and created menswear with elegant fluidity of movement and, ultimately, an androgynous look.

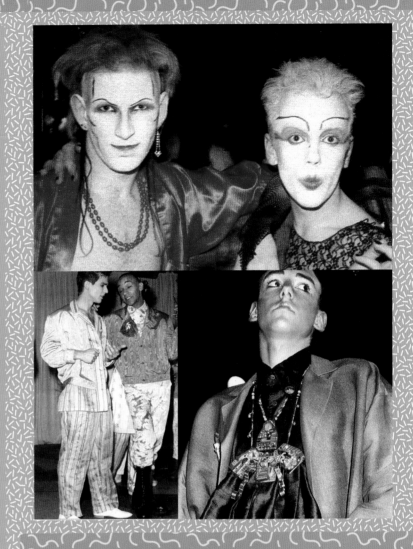

SUITED AND BOOTED

Heavy media influence throughout the decade resulted in no particular suit style reigning supreme. In fact, the eighties saw a mix and match in suit cuts and fabrics from past decades. Contemporary designers of the day were creating less structured fits with innovative detailing, such as risqué buttons or odd-shaped lapels, and with unusual pattern cutting and irregular hemlines for an unconventional fit on the body. Tuxedo fashions followed the same trend with slimmer-fitting cuts worn by the younger generation and more traditional, looser, double-breasted versions worn by senior gentlemen.

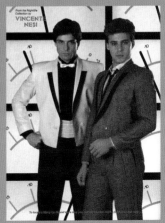

1980s SHOES

During the previous decade designers had started to expand the boundaries of fashion with surprising results for footwear design. The end of the seventies had given both men and women variety in practical shoes as well as the opportunity to wear something a little more interesting on their feet if they desired. The distinction between men's and women's shoes was becoming less obvious as trends moved away from gender-defined fashion, instead giving the wearer an opportunity to experiment as they pleased.

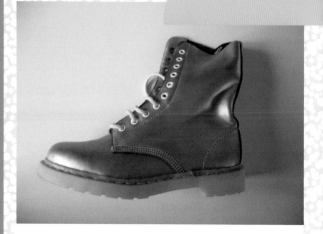

DOCTOR DOCTOR.....

If Klaus Martens hadn't sustained an injury during the World War II, it is possible that the iconic Dr Martens footwear we know and love today might never have been invented. The ox-blood, air-cushioned-sole boot was synonymous with the eighties, and had ties to skinhead culture, post punk and the Hard Times look.

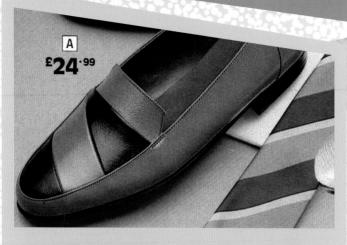

A
£24·⁹⁹

LOAFING AROUND

The loafer slip-on began as a casual house shoe back in the mid-1800s, and was famously made a key part of Gucci's signature shoe collection in 1953. Its evolution into unisex smart casual footwear can be seen if we fast forward to the eighties. Adopted by Preppies and New Romantics alike, the loafer was worn with trousers, jeans, skirts and suits.

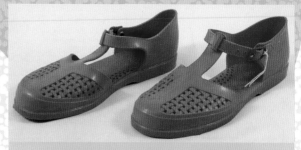

JELLY ON THE BEACH

It would be impossible to talk about eighties fashion without mentioning jelly shoes. The plastic footwear has undefined origins, with speculation about the first designs going right back to World War II, but it is undisputed that they were all the rage in the eighties.

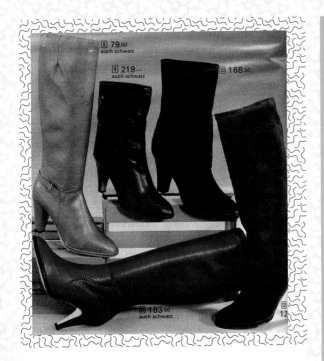

KNEE DEEP

The knee-high boot was a popular choice during the decade and often extended above the knee to the thigh for those looking for a more fetish/Gothic style. Worn predominantly by women during the eighties this footwear wasn't gender exclusive and variations were sometimes associated with heavy metal and rock subcultures.

TRAINING HARD

Trainers, or sneakers as they are referred to Stateside, were the ultimate fashion statement in the eighties. It wasn't a prerequisite to participate in sport while wearing them. It was simply cool to have the latest 'must have' pair, and there was considerable choice to pick from. Nike seemed to rule the roost for the most part with their Air Jordan, Air Force, Dunk and Air Max ranges, but there was significant competition in the form of Converse Weapon and Adidas Decade, as well as British brands like Reebok, which launched its popular women's Freestyle range in 1982.

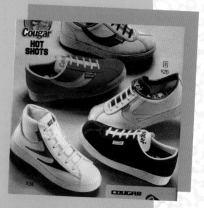

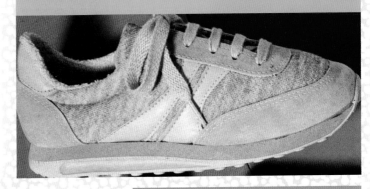

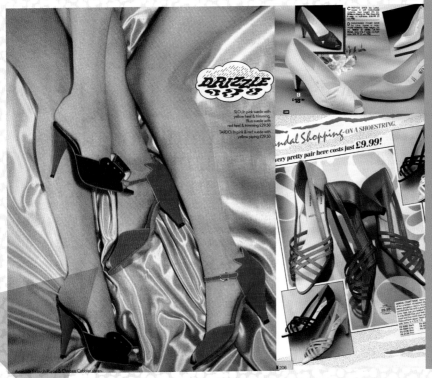

ORDER IN COURT

As with most other fashions, there were huge variations in the footwear women chose to wear, but the consensus for up-to-the-moment sexy footwear was the mid-heel court shoe. More often than not, the eighties court shoe would be bold in colour, and sometimes also pattern, with a rounded, slightly pointed toe, high sides and a cone shape mid-heel, around 7.5cm (3 in) high. Other heel types popular on a court shoe included the prism and the kitten heel.

1980s SPORTSWEAR

By the 1980s, the consumer market for sportswear wasn't targeted just at those wanting to engage in physical activity, it was now fundamental to fashion in its own right. The craze for sport and in particular fitness during the eighties meant that established sportswear and leisurewear brands were able to target those individuals wanting to be part of a fashion subculture as well as those hitting the gym.

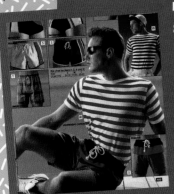

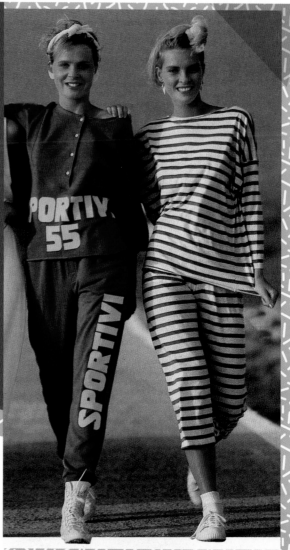

REMEMBER MY NAME...FAME!

As a French trapeze artist in the 1800s, it was imperative for Jules Leotard to wear an outfit that did not restrict his movement and which also allowed him to show off his impressive physique. And so a garment was born – one that was to epitomize a casual look nearly two hundred years later. By the 1980s it was the likes of the TV show *Fame* that had brought the leotard into the forefront of fashion. A precursor for the 'body' in the nineties, the spandex or Lycra leotard was worn for exercising as well as in casual fashion ensembles.

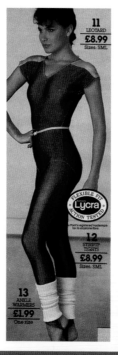

11
LEOTARD
£8.99
Sizes: SML

12
STIRRUP
TIGHTS
£8.99
Sizes: SML

13
ANKLE
WARMERS
£1.99
One size

JUMPING THROUGH HOOPS

The eighties was a decade obsessed with basketball and the footwear associated with it. When US player Michael Jordan staked his claim to be the best basketball player to have ever lived, athletic companies clamoured for his endorsement. It was Nike that won the contract, branding their iconic range of trainers with MJ's nickname – 'Air Jordan'.

DANCING THE NIGHT AWAY

Leg warmers were originally used by dancers as a means of keeping lower leg muscles warm, but like the leotard they were adopted as a general fashion trend in the eighties. More often than not, leg warmers were knitted, although variations in fabric evolved as they became a general fashion item.

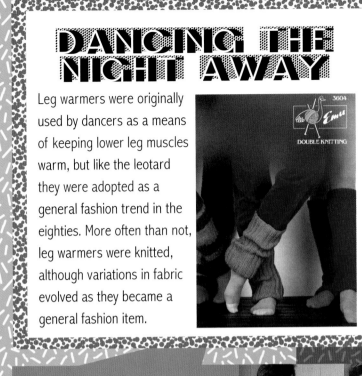

YOU CANNOT BE SERIOUS!

Tennis had its fair share of characters in the eighties, most notably famously bad-tempered John McEnroe, but it was Swede Björn Borg who was setting sportswear standards with his affiliation to Fila. By the eighties the craze for keeping fit or at least looking sporty made tennis apparel appealing both on and off court. At the start of the decade, Fila launched the Settanta Mk2 in three colours – navy blue, light blue and red. The Terrinda Mk3 was brought out in 1982 with a biker-style collar and padded shoulder detail, however this was to be the last Fila BJ tracksuit top.

TRACK-SUITED & BOOTED

The tracksuit or leisure suit had well and truly evolved to become part of the circus of fashion by the eighties with Adidas, Reebok and Ellesse among the leading brands in demand. Although worn by both sexes, it was menswear that really embraced the style, making it an acceptable means of casual wear for almost all non-formal occasions, including evening wear for raves and hip-hop clubs.

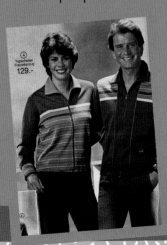

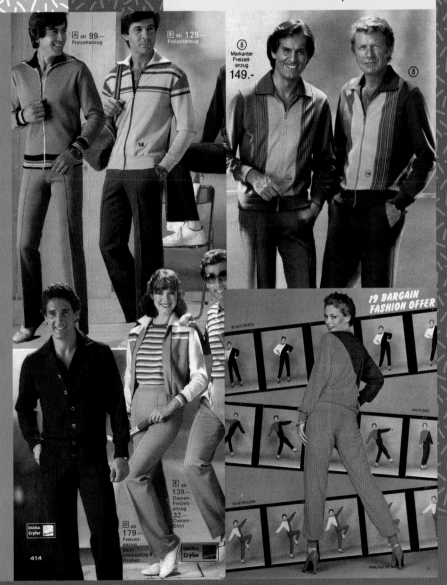

1980s ACCESSORIES

The trend for excess was never easier to achieve than with the accessories of the eighties! Almost all leading designers had expanded their clothing collections to accommodate the growing demand from consumers to own items with a desirable 'label', meaning that even if you couldn't afford the haute couture clothes, you could own designer accessories.

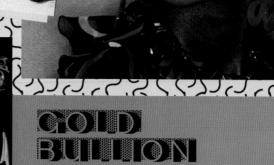

GOLD BULLION

Gold was the all-pervasive theme of jewellery during the decade, with the precious-metal colour signifying opulence and success. Many of the leading design houses like Chanel, Versace, Dior and Moschino presented chunky faux-gold costume jewellery ranges with diamanté and faux pearls. These were quickly copied by high-street retailers for a fraction of the cost. This trend didn't stop at jewellery though, it extended to all accessories including belts, bags and sunglasses.

TIME FOR CHANGE

The quartz revolution in the late seventies and eighties saw the demise of traditional Swiss watch manufacture and the rise in popularity of quartz watches. The first twelve models of Swatch watch designs were released in 1983, proving to be an instant hit. The Pop Swatch allowed the wearer to change the main face of the watch and even attach it directly to clothing, making this one of the most popular accessories of the decade with both young and old.

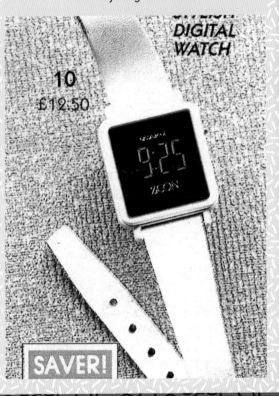

GHETTO BLASTERS

Admittedly not strictly a fashion item, ghetto blasters were worn on the shoulder so prolifically during the decade, it would be a shame to overlook them as the ultimate eighties accessory! If you don't fancy carrying one around with you, consider a ghetto-blaster set of earrings or necklace to pay homage to the trend.

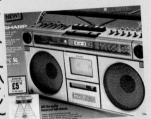

GET THE LOOK WITH HANNAH

The classic 2.55 quilted Chanel flap bag, so called as it was originally launched in February 1955, was considered the ultimate symbol of success in the eighties. The bag comes in a variety of sizes and looks as good with casual clothing as it does with a little black dress. Make sure you know the tell-tale signs of the genuine article to avoid parting with cash for a fake.

BOY OH BOY

Madonna and Boy George were among some of the high-profile pop stars creating fashion waves alongside their music. Their respective signature looks caused controversy among many who felt their provocative and gender-bending fashion statements were a step too far for their eighties audiences. Despite this, their fashion style, which consisted of bows and lace and lots and lots of jewellery, struck a chord with millions of young men and women who immediately took to replicating it by wearing make-up, hats, leather wrist cuffs, crucifixes and layer upon layer of silver chains.

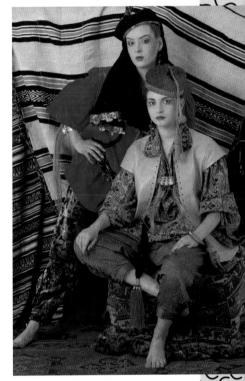

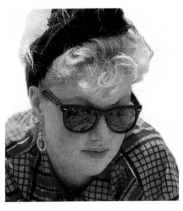

1980s GET THE LOOK WITH HANNAH

Y ou can have a lot of fun experimenting with achieving an authentic eighties look. The decade encompassed bright colours and big hair for both sexes, which can be taken to the extreme should you want to. The diversity of style that the decade produced means that there will be something for everyone and you should play around with what works best for you.

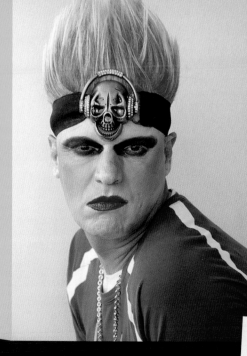

BRIGHT EYES

Blue and purple eye shadow replace the earthy browns of the seventies and can be worn for both day and evening looks. Don't worry about sticking to the socket area — eighties styles were much more theatrical! These colours extend to the lips too, but use a matching lip liner (or eyeliner if you can't match the colour) to give precision to the outer edge of your lips. Varying shades of pink dominate blusher palettes, with a trend for heavy application, so try smiling and placing the blush on the apples of your cheeks in a circular motion and then sweeping diagonally up towards your hairline. Repeat until you have achieved the depth of colour required.

HAIR FLAIR

Endless variety marked hair styling in the eighties. Before you attempt a signature style, decide how permanent you want your look to be. The high-top afro was worn naturally and shaped accordingly, as was the bobbed undercut, but both of these styles require regular maintenance. Crimping can be done at home with a crimping tool, but use a heat protector spray before you start to avoid damaging your hair.

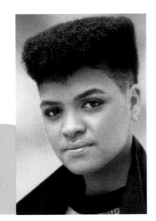

HIGH VOLUME

Volume is best achieved on hair that has been freshly washed, and ideally it should be cut in layers. Towel dry and apply a volume-enhancing mousse or root spray. Bend over and rough dry your hair upside down. When it feels dry, flip your hair back. Using a pintail comb, backcomb the crown area. Warm a little wax on your fingertips by rubbing your hands together, then separate the layers, teasing upwards and outwards. When you are happy, hairspray into place.

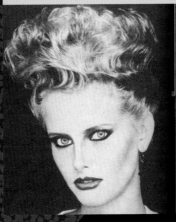
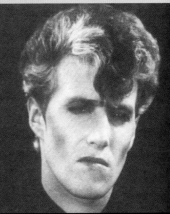

UPTOWN PUNK

Full-on punk fashion can be too edgy for most, but it can be dipped into. Vintage Vivienne Westwood costume jewellery is unisex and highly collectable. Ladies can add a touch of punk by combining a black leather or PVC pencil skirt with a plain black chunky-knit jumper. Asymmetric necklines or oversized jumpers that fall off one shoulder will expose a bra strap, which can be customized to add a delicate punk twist by stitching or sticking (using fabric glue) some tartan ribbon onto the exposed strap. You can further accessorize the jumper with a kilt-pin 'brooch'.

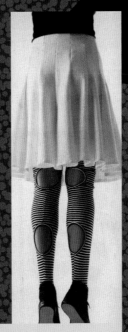

BRACES

A unisex and great way to add interest to your outfit, braces come in a variety of colours — black can be quite striking but look out for softer greens, browns and beiges, too. If you are buying vintage braces, you may need to add buttons to the inside of your trouser waistband.

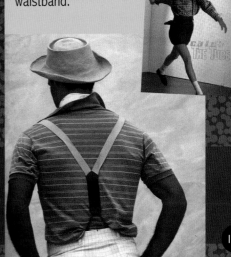

TIGHT EMBRACE

Tights were overtaking stockings as a more popular choice of hosiery in the eighties. Team large-pattern fishnets in black or red with mid-heel court shoes for a sexy night time look or for a funky and fun daytime attire, try striped 40+ denier opaques.

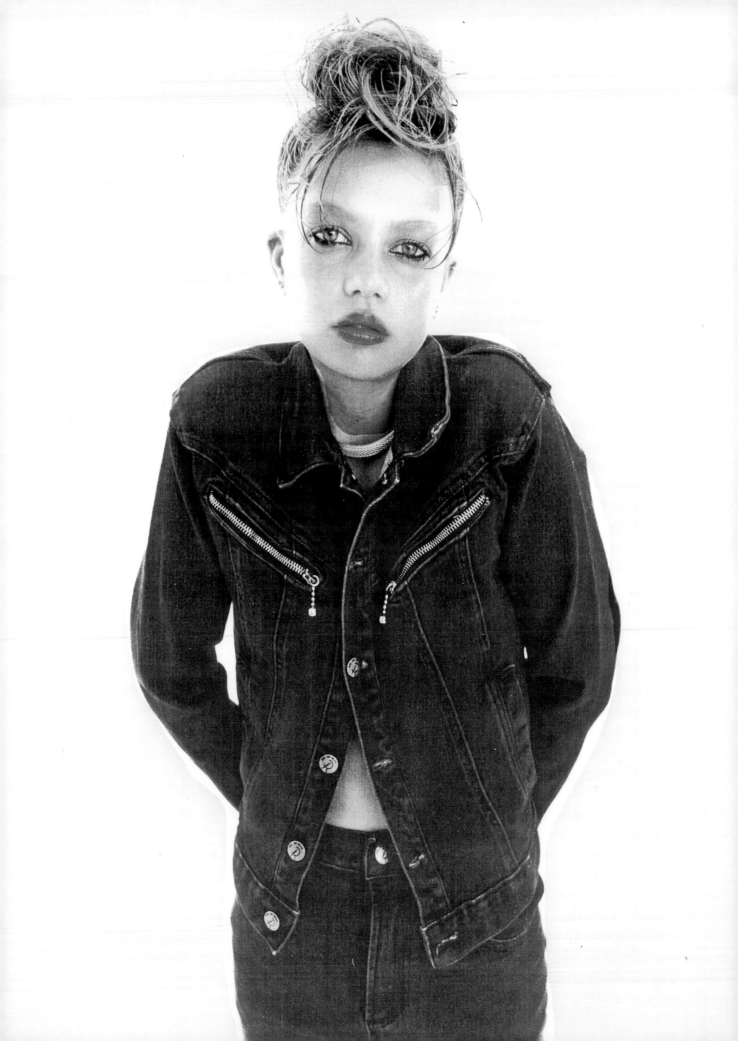

As a decade only recently considered 'vintage' the nineties is proving to be a significant period in fashion history, one which conjured up a hotchpotch of styles and adopted an almost 'anything goes' way of thinking. New blood and alternative fashion notions disregarded the necessity to appeal to a broad audience, instead focusing on conceptual design and 'intelligent' fashion, which would connect with specific groups. As a consequence, the fashion industry followed a new path which would reset the bar for innovative, quirky and often downright controversial ensembles. This new passion would flow through the veins of the industry and dominate the fashion headlines.

Body shape and size remained integral to showcasing the cut of clothing. The previous decade's obsession with fitness had focussed on models with lean muscle mass, and had seen the introduction of athletic and Amazonian supermodels treading the catwalk. However, at the start of the nineties the fashion elite, striving for a point of difference, presented collections on models at the opposite end of the body-shape spectrum. They created new interest, but also caused much controversy, with pale and emaciated models in a trend that was dubbed 'heroin chic'. In 1990, self-taught fashion photographer Corrine Day photographed a 16-year-old Kate Moss for an editorial spread for *Face* magazine. Three years later, Moss and her waif-like frame were hot property and Day was shooting with her at the model's flat for a front cover of *Vogue*.

Those images were the catalyst for the subsequent androgynous designs that filled the catwalks, presented on models with no body fat, whose razorp-sharp bone structure was highlighted by exposed décolletage and hips. The trend meant that haute couture fashion was being geared towards a body size that was simply unobtainable for the majority of high-street shoppers. With the top fashion houses providing the bedrock for mainstream high-street design, heroin chic was slammed by press and public opinion alike for glamorizing an unhealthy body image, dangerous lifestyle choices and even an unacceptable interest in pre-pubescent bodies. In 1997, when heroin chic was at its peak, 13 designers including John Galliano, Stella McCartney, John Rocha, Reynold Pearce and Andrew Fionda made a statement in protest: 'We disapprove of the fashion industry glamorizing the use of addictive substances as this could have a detrimental effect on the lives of young people, many of whom are greatly influenced by the appearance and actions of members of our industry.' The initial chatter around the trend escalated its appeal but faded toward the end of the decade, although controversy about models' body shape and size remained.

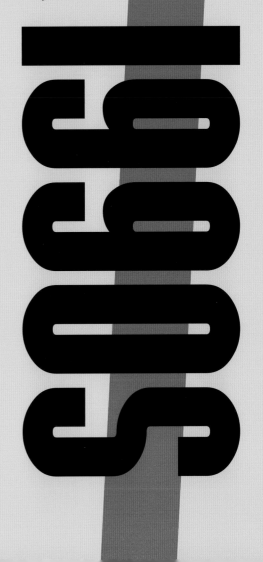

1990S MEN & WOMEN'S WEAR

Pulp, The Charlatans, Happy Mondays, The Stone Roses, Inspiral Carpets and Ocean Colour Scene were among a vast scene of musicians who played a dramatic part in shaping nineties fashion in the UK and abroad. The popularity and appeal of Brit Pop meant that band followers channelled specific looks. In Britain there was a north/south divide between Oasis and Blur, with the northern Gallagher brothers choosing thigh-length parka coats, baggy-fit jeans, Argyle jumpers, polo shirts and Adidas Gazelle trainers. In the south, Blur borrowed elements of the 1950s, popularizing tartan-lined Harrington jackets and Levi jeans. Elastica and Suede couple Justine Frischmann and Brett Anderson went for a more traditional 'rock star' look with a combo of dark skinny jeans and cropped leather jacket. All of these looks were identified as a 'Cool Britannia' uniform which would become characteristic of the nineties image. Even new British designers like Alice Temperley, Hussein Chalayan and Matthew Williamson looked to the past to shape collections for the future. The British bands that dominated the charts popularized old-school brands such as Fred Perry and Ben Sherman as well as celebrating recently established brands like Nigel Hall, Hope & Glory and Duffer of St George.

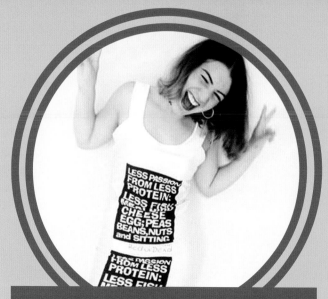

MAKING A STATEMENT

The slogan T-shirt of the seventies had given way to fashion followers wearing logos and labels on the outside so it was only a matter of time before politics, religion and lifestyle choices made their way onto and into our clothes. Many designers had strong ethical opinions on manufacturing processes, materials and political agendas. With the internet granting individuals 24-hour access to injustice around the globe, it was only a matter of time before fashion allowed designers to earn a reputation as much for their ethics as for the cut of their cloth.

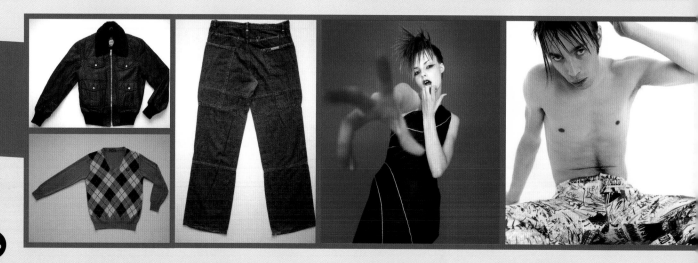

GET THE GRIME

The nineties gave us grunge – a subculture whose fashion ideology borrowed from heavy metal, rock and punk and whose followers listened to music from the likes of Nirvana and Pearl Jam. The hardcore grunge followers adopted the 'dirt and grime' definition of the word, choosing loose fitting T-shirts, jeans, biker jackets and patterned jumpers. The more 'soft grungers' chose to expand their colour and style palette, mixing stone-wash or acid-wash denim, Dr Marten boots or brightly-coloured trainers with plaid flannel shirts.

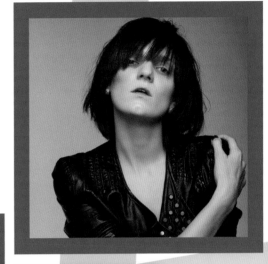

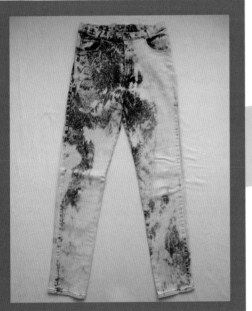

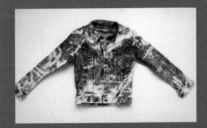

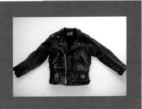

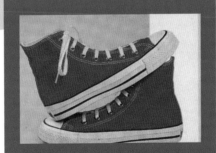

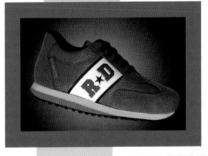

FLORAL *NATION*

Nature provided the inspiration for a nineties fad for floral shirts. A unisex trend, the shirts ranged from slim-fit to oversized and came in a variety of blooms. The Liberty Arts fabric collection had been selling floral material since 1870 and the rise in its popularity meant that floral shirts appealed to a variety of fashion followers, including soft grungers and ravers. The botanical reference was also adopted by British designer Paul Smith, who liked to hide floral detailing on the inside of his creations as well as using it on the outside of his designs.

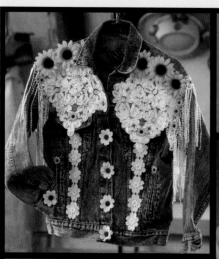

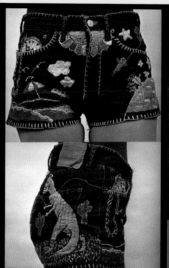

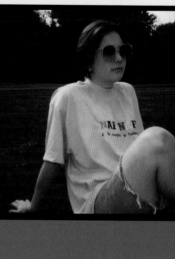

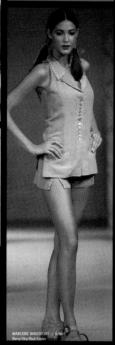

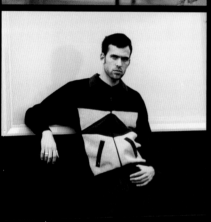

MARLENE WAISCOAT – S/M/L
Navy/Sky/Red/Green

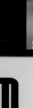

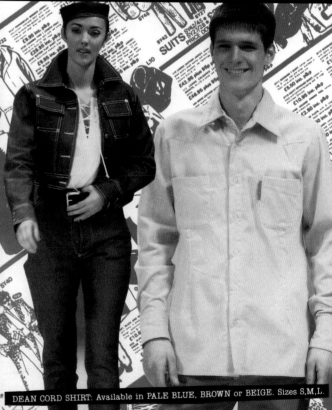

DEAN CORD SHIRT: Available in PALE BLUE, BROWN or BEIGE. Sizes S,M,L.

SUTTON MENS TROUSERS: Available in DENIM or TOBACCO. Sizes S,M,L.

WORKWEAR

P.J. WOMENS JACKET: Available in DENIM or TOBACCO. Sizes S,M,L.

LINDA WOMENS TROUSERS: Available in DENIM or TOBACCO. Sizes S,M,L.

DENIM

Denim remained a strong player in nineties fashion. Owing to relaxed ideas about what consituted day and evening wear, and the versitility of the fabric, it featured in all fashion areas. The beauty of denim construction allows for a light and heavyweight weave, and fashion played with this to create new textures, with the addition of Elastane and Lycra for extra stretch. Levis continued to dominate the market in the nineties and there was a big trend for worn and embellished denim, boosting the success of second-hand markets in places like Camden in north London.

BLACK *MAGIC*

Wearing black, gold and a splash of red was almost mandatory during the nineties. The decade was swamped with designer brands, and the classic combination of these three colours became heavily associated with Italian brand Moschino and its Cheap & Chic range. The company had been established in the late eighties by Franco Moschino, who aimed to satirize fashion with its take on gaudy big-name brand designs. It was quite ironic when Moschino's success turned it into a big-name fashion brand in its own right.

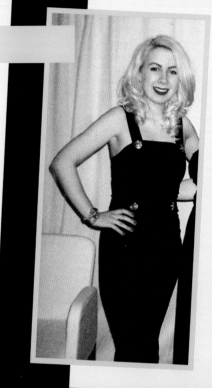

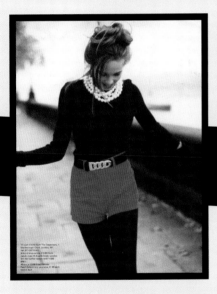

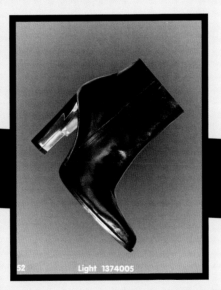

52   Light 1374005

RETRO CELEBRATION

From crop tops to flares, frills to tartan, the catwalks and high streets were awash with nods to the past. Nineties collections were peppered with sixties and seventies styles, creating focal points of interest from past decades.

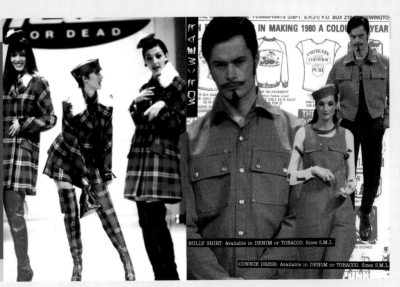

BULLY SHIRT: Available in DENIM or TOBACCO. Sizes S,M,L.

CONNIE DRESS: Available in DENIM or TOBACCO. Sizes S,M,L.

Funk 'n' Sole

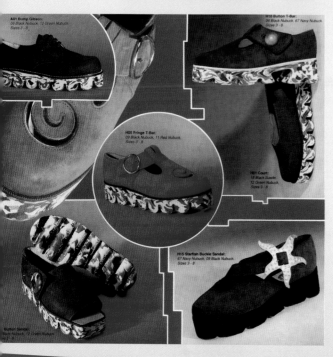

A01 Bump Gibson:
09 Black Nubuck, 12 Green Nubuck
Sizes 3 - 8

H10 Button T-Bar:
06 Black Nubuck, 67 Navy Nubuck
Sizes 3 - 8

H05 Fringe T-Bar:
09 Black Nubuck, 11 Red Nubuck
Sizes 3 - 8

H01 Court:
18 Black Suede,
12 Green Nubuck
Sizes 3 - 8

H15 Starfish Buckle Sandal:
67 Navy Nubuck, 09 Black Nubuck
Sizes 3 - 8

Button Sandal:
Black Nubuck, 12 Green Nubuck

Shoe styles available for both men and women had evolved over the decades, with a plentiful selection on offer by the nineties, but designers still looked to push the fashion boundaries. Alternative materials like foam were being used to create lightweight, platform-based shoes and sandals with deep ridged soles. These shoes proved a big hit on the rave scene with their colourful patterned soles, and were also a firm favourite alongside wellington boots on the festival scene. Espadrilles, too, gained popularity during the decade, with both men and women wearing them.

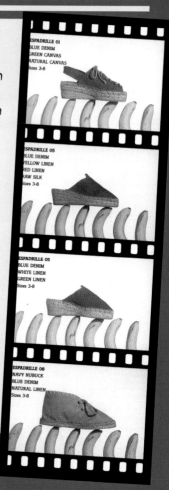

ESPADRILLE 01
BLUE DENIM
GREEN CANVAS
NATURAL CANVAS
Sizes 3-8

ESPADRILLE 05
BLUE DENIM
YELLOW LINEN
RED LINEN
RAW SILK
Sizes 3-8

ESPADRILLE 05
BLUE DENIM
WHITE LINEN
GREEN LINEN
Sizes 3-8

ESPADRILLE 08
NAVY NUBUCK
BLUE DENIM
NATURAL LINEN
Sizes 3-8

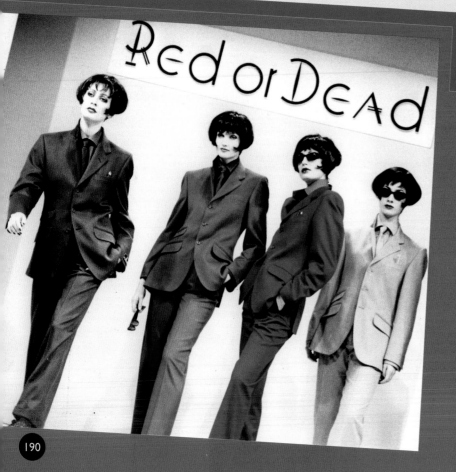

SUIT CASE

The cut of suits for both sexes became almost identical in the nineties, with both men and women electing to wear shirts, ties, waistcoats and trousers. The single-breasted, three-button suit with flap pockets and trouser cuffs provided a classic look that was adopted by city workers as well as those looking for formal occasion attire. In terms of fabric choices, colour and pattern palettes varied from bright and bold, to pastel and subtle. Outside of formal wear, both men and women teamed smart suit jackets with chinos or denim for a somewhere-in-between 'smart casual' look.

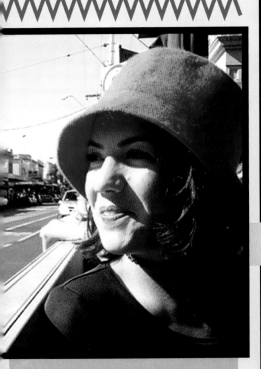

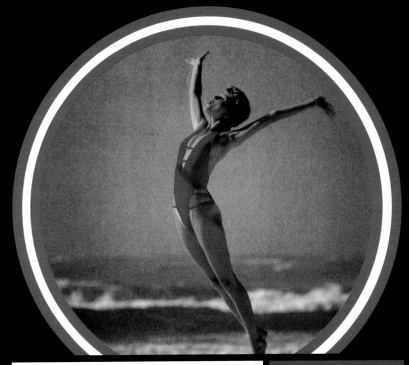

CHOKERS

Wearing chokers is most commonly asssociated with high fashion during the Victorian era, when a black velvet ribbon would be decorated with filigree silver or cameo detailing. This trend made a comeback in the nineties, with plastic, metal, fabric and leather featuring gemstones and spikes among other decorations. Easy to create at home, chokers showcased an eclectic mix of ribbons and woven thread and could even be knitted.

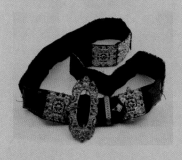

PASS THE REMOTE

Television had become central to the majority of homes by the 1990s, and many households owned more than one set. This, coupled with the hundreds of channels available via satellite dishes, gave UK audiences access to a wide variety of programmes from around the world. *Baywatch*, *Friends* and *Beverly Hills 90210* created trends for skimpy swimwear, slip dresses, chinos, blazers and tube dresses. *Sex and the City* in particular gained notoriety for the clothing of its four main characters, with designs by such greats as Manolo Blahnik and Vivienne Westwood making regular appearances as the show's wardrobe mixed couture, high-street and customized styling effortlessly.

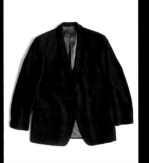

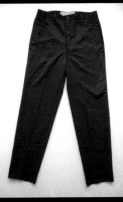

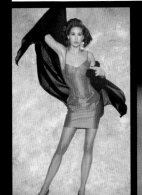

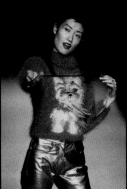

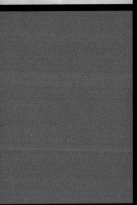

1990s GET THE LOOK WITH HANNAH

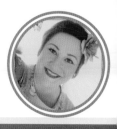

Experimenting was 'cool' in the nineties, creating temporary fads as well as more iconic looks. Make-up and hairstyles were heavily influenced by music subcultures so try twisting sections of hair into knotted buns all over your head (Gwen Stefani/Bjork) or use miniature butterfly clips to hold channelled sections of hair away from your face and add lots and lots of hair glitter. In an era when fake tan was yet to hit the shops, skin was almost always pale and provided a stark contrast to smoky kohl-lined eyes and dark red lips. The crop top was huge on the rave scene so show off toned stomachs with high-waisted shorts or Lycra skirts. For the ultimate place to get your raving wardrobe, visit Cyberdog; its roots were established in the heart of London's Camden Market in 1994.

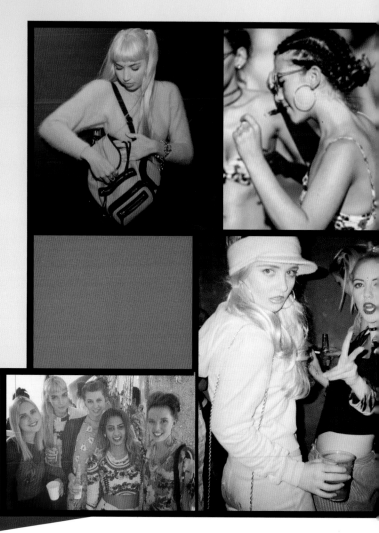

ZIGZAG PARTINGS

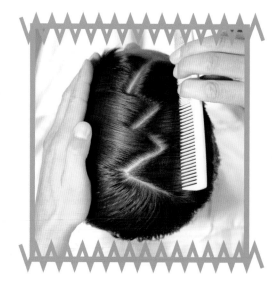

Zigzag hair partings are a simple and effective way to create a nineties look. Opt to zigzag all the way through or only for some of the parting. Make sure your hair isn't too flyaway by using a small amount of serum and then, using either a pintail comb or medium-sized straight comb, mark the first part of your parting. Change direction and mark the next bit of your parting, ensuring that you sweep all the hair from that particular section in the opposite direction. Repeat this until your chosen size parting is in a zigzag shape. It's a flexible style - you can make the parting as small and intricate or large and bold as you like!

HAIR RAISING

Seemingly not wanting to be left out of the hair mania that swept the nineties, the gents took to growing theirs into 'curtains'. This involves growing your hair all over to one length, or alternatively growing just the top section over the crown and keeping the sides and back closely shaved. The long hair should then be parted, like curtains, in the centre.

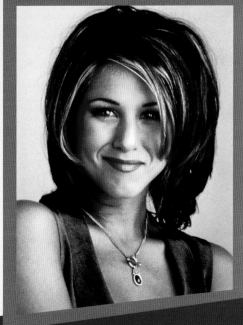

THE RACHEL

Jennifer Aniston's long, layered bouncy bob was created by Chris McMillan for her *Friends* character, Rachel Green (left), and to recreate it will require a visit to the hairdresser to add choppy layers into shoulder-length hair. Using a good root-lift mousse and large rounded brush with a high-speed hairdryer will allow you to maintain this look.

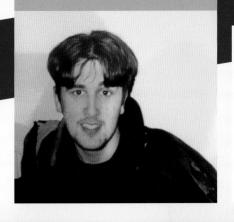

FLASHING YA PANTS

Bare chests, six packs (not the alcohol variety) with just a hint of Calvin Klein underpants above baggy jeans was not only considered cool, but positively sexy in the nineties, so dust off your gym membership card and unleash your inner Peter André!

LIPPY LADIES

For the ultimate nineties make-up look, seek out a plum or dark cherry shade of lipstick. This colour can be difficult to wear so it is vital that your lips aren't dry or chapped and it's just as important to find a suitable lip liner to make sure that the shape is perfect.

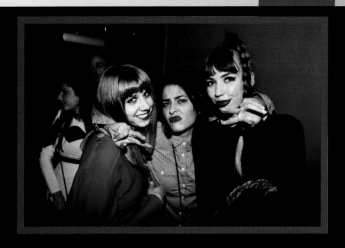

FUTURE
VINTAGE

Fashion in the 'noughties' and beyond has been a fusion of vintage styles, traditional ethnic wear and art. Catwalk shows have become as much about the creativity in showcasing new collections as the collections themselves. In an industry famed for pushing boundaries, recent designs have reached new heights of creativity and will undoubtedly go on to become regarded as future vintage. Here is a small selection of designers that are highly collectable and items and fashion trends that we think may be what vintage fans will be wearing in years to come.

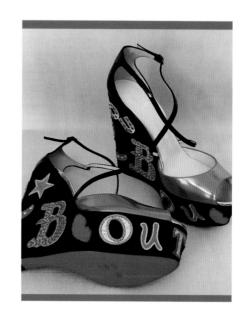

Christian Louboutin

Louboutin's signature red-soled shoes have become synonymous with sexiness and style. Starting out with his first store in the early 1990s in Paris, the brand focused almost entirely on the elegance of the stiletto and how it changed the way a woman carried herself. Louboutin celebrated his 20th anniversary in 2011 and has expanded his designs into handbags and nail polish as well as men's shoes.

Alexander McQueen

The designer's untimely death in 2010 shocked the fashion world. Renowned for his controversial designs and use of shock tactics, McQueen's signature was the skull, incorporated onto scarves, shoes, bags and wallets. His bumster trousers, featured in his first collection, were an ultra low-rise creation – he declared the bottom of the spine to be most erotic – and were to be the start of collections peppered with fetish and references to death. The brand continues today under the creative direction of McQueen's former assistant, Sarah Burton.

Anya Hindmarch

Famed for her 'Be a Bag' range, popular with celebrities, Hindmarch collaborated with the global social change movement Shift (formerly known as We Are What We Do) in 2007 to create a shopping tote alternative to plastic carrier bags. They were a strictly limited edition and retailed for £5; however, it sold out almost instantly, and the bags were being traded for prices in excess of £150 within days.

Stella McCartney

Graduating from prestigious Central Saint Martins in 1995, Stella McCartney interned at Christian Lacroix and fine-tuned her skills as a designer working for Edward Sexton. When she launched her first collection, it came as no surprise to see sassy designs detailed with top-class tailoring. In 1997, McCartney was appointed the Creative Director of Chloé in Paris. She is a staunch vegetarian and supporter of PETA and refuses to use leather and fur in her designs.

Paul Smith

Paul Smith's quirky and elegant brand features clothes, shoes and accessories for men, women and children as well as a limited range of homeware. His 'Men Only' shoe range for women echoes the men's mainline collection. His floral designs reflect his passion for gardening and the brand is noted for collections in his signature stripe.

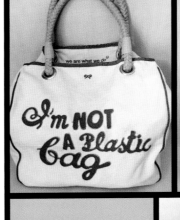
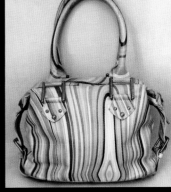
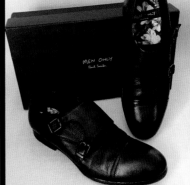

[clockwise from top left] Anya Hindmarch tote; a trio of Paul Smith designs – a handbag in his signature stripe, his 'Men Only' Keaton shoes for women, and a floral canvas bag; Christian Louboutin Loubi Zeppa clutch bag, matching shoes opposite.

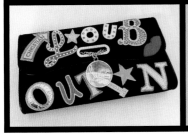
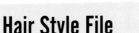

Hair Style File

These are the hairstyles that will complete the vintage look of the future:

The Lob - A long bob hairstyle cut just above the shoulders. Can work on layered hair or one length.

The Undercut - Trendy for men and women, the undercut requires long hair on top with either one or both sides shaved down typically to a grade 1 (clipper length).

Dip-Dyed Hair - Sometimes referred to as the Ombre, this trend was popular among women who dye the lower half of their mid-length to long hair in a contrasting colour.

Fishtail Plaits - Intricate braiding that requires hair to be crossed over from two wide sections of hair. Usually worn low down on the sides of the head.

Rainbow Hair - Hair dyed in a rainbow of colours and worn poker straight with a light serum or hairspray.

Top Knots - A unisex trend where long hair is tied into a knot on the top of the head.

Hipster Beards - Large fisherman-style beards and often large side burns which would typically be sported with a totally shaved head or top knot.

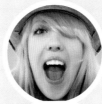
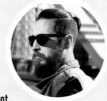

Tattoos

Not a new phenomenon, tattoos and tattoo designs have fallen in and out fashion over the years. Tribal, sailor and Mexican 'día de los muertos' are among some of the most popular in the noughties. Transfers will work just as well for that future vintage noughties party.

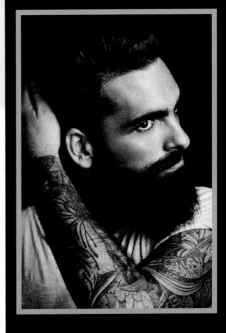

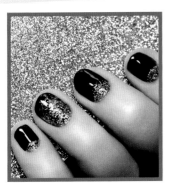

Nail Art

With a trend for intricate designs, brands like Minx offered temporary nail art on transfer sheets which could be heated and applied instantly. When those requiring more durability from their polish spoke out, long-lasting and unchippable polishes were created by brands like Bio-Gel and Shellac. Stock up on these for an authentic future vintage look.

BUYING VINTAGE

Sale TIME

The key to successful vintage clothes shopping is to take a look at your body shape and take accurate measurements. Write them down and keep them with you. Armed with your measurements, take a mental note of the parts of your body you want to show off and cross reference this with fashion trends that will suit you best. There is no hard and fast rule that you have to embrace a particular era in its entirety so pick and choose accordingly.

Underwear

Underwear plays a crucial part in how a garment looks. Over the years, men moved from large boxer shorts and long johns to Y-fronts, and ladies sported bullet bras, girdles, bust-flattening bras and waist cinchers to help mould their shape to fit the fashion. If you don't get your foundation garments right, it is unlikely those drainpipe trousers or wiggle dress will sit correctly on the body.

$1/11\frac{1}{2}$

1! 8ᴰ 1!

Get charted!

For a handy measurements checklist, use a costume measurement chart – there are many available online. It will include all areas of your body from head to foot. Keep this list up to date.

Taped

Always carry a fabric tape measure in your handbag when you go shopping. This will allow you to measure clothes and shoes and save you trying on every single item in the shop.

NOW 1/3

Leather looks

Check vintage leather for signs of cracking. If the leather has become brittle and hard it will break when stressed. Gently bend back the sole of a shoe to test how supple it is or place a light weight inside a bag to test the handle. Ask the person you are buying from to do these tests to avoid landing the bill for ruining stock!

Worn out

Always consider the condition of the item you are buying and weigh up whether any damage can be repaired easily. Bear in mind that a lot of vintage fashion wasn't made to be worn for vigorous activities.

1! DOWN

Size wise

When shopping online, obtain the measurements for the item rather than asking for the size. This is important for men and women but sizes for women's clothes in particular have altered dramatically over the last 80 years. A size 16 woman's dress from the 1960s would probably fit a modern-day size 12, and clothing from this period rarely had a sizing label as standard. As now, there was also a varying scale used in different countries so a US size 10 would be a UK size 14. Knowing your measurements and asking for clarification will save you disappointment.

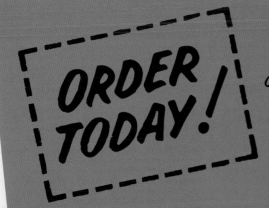

ORDER TODAY!

Hang ups!

Check the inside of the shoulders on vintage garments to make sure they don't have small tears or rust marks caused by using the wrong clothes hangers. Padded hangers are a must for delicate garments and heavy wool as they will stop the item becoming misshapen.

Quality v Quantity

Buying second hand should allow you to get more for your money in most cases as vintage clothing will usually be better made and higher quality compared to modern clothing. Build a capsule wardrobe that can be mixed and matched and aim for quality over quantity as you will get more wear out of the items in the long run.

Vintage clothing stores are always looking for new stock so consider trading in some of your unwanted items for replacement pieces.

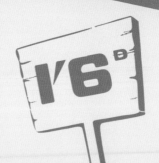

Prices aren't always fixed on vintage items so try negotiating for a wanted item.

Smell check!

Check the lining in jackets and trousers as this may have torn, which can cause garments to hang badly or stick where they shouldn't! As crude as it might seem, don't forget to check the crotch and armpits of vintage clothing as it may not be possible to remove stains or smells.

Fake alert!

Faking labels like Chanel and Dior is big business. If you collect designer pieces, familiarize yourself with the brand and watch out for poor-quality materials, buttons and zips as well as amateur stitching. If you are thinking of investing in a pre-loved designer item it's worth doing your homework and, if possible, getting authentication from a specialist site or direct from the design house itself.

Timeless chic

Whether you are starting a vintage fashion collection or simply adding to an existing one, you can't go wrong by buying basic, classic pieces. Items like a little black dress or a white shirt, black stilettos or a trilby hat won't lose their appeal and can be mixed and matched with other vintage items or clothes in your contemporary wardrobe.

24'11 OR ONLY 3'6 DOWN

Perfume can tarnish costume jewellery so check for signs of discolouration, especially on necklaces and bracelets, and take care when spraying scent yourself.

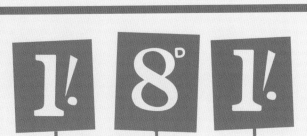

1'. 8ᴰ 1'.

18'11 VALUE FOR ONLY 9'11 1'- DOWN 2'- MONTH

Shoe store

Check how shoes are being sold; if they are all thrown into a box this could cause scuffing and scratching. Also, they should not be kept in direct sunlight, as this can cause fading. Look for shoes that have shoe stretchers or tissue paper to minimize creases. To care for your shoes at home, clean them regularly and allow them to dry properly. Rubber soles and metal caps will prolong the life of shoes as will using a good leather moisturizer or suede brush and protector.

ASK THE EXPERT

Collecting Vintage

Holly Foster, a 22-year-old office worker, wears vintage clothes almost every day. She has been a collector of vintage fashion for the last few years.

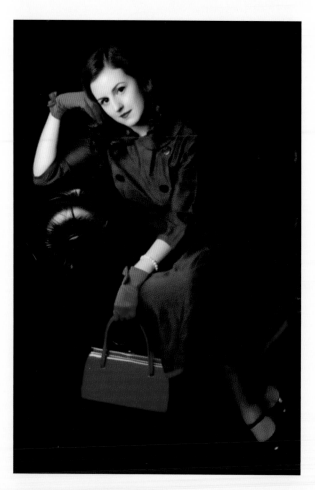

When did you first start collecting vintage fashion and why?

I first started collecting vintage at the age of fifteen when I made my first purchase at a charity shop in my local town. It was a 1960s crimplene shift dress with little purple flowers – nothing really elegant or pretty. However, a week later I returned and bought a beautiful pair of yellow driving gloves. Thus my affair with vintage began.

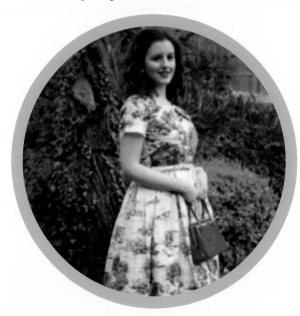

How large is your personal vintage fashion collection and what does it consist of?

I would say I have about 150 to 200 pieces of vintage in my wardrobe, most of which I wear on a daily basis. My collection consists mainly of dresses, sweaters and skirts. I adore the 1950s styles and collect a rare label called California Cottons amongst other designers like Jonathan Logan. More recently I've started collecting novelty prints, which are great fun.

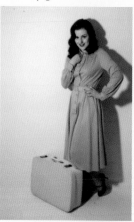
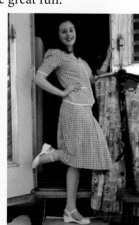

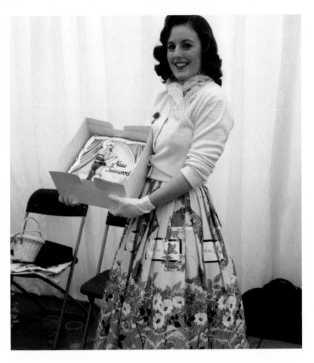

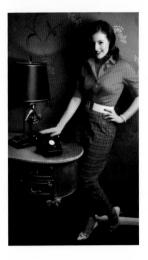

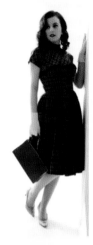

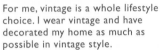

For me, vintage is a whole lifestyle choice. I wear vintage and have decorated my home as much as possible in vintage style.

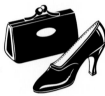

What are our favourite items?

I have an unworn 1950s sweater that I purchased from a secret group on Facebook, designed by Harry M Goodstein for St Laurent. It is pink with pearl beading in the shape of a bow and I adore it. It came in the original packaging, all sealed in pink tissue paper. I also have a Lana Lobell novelty print skirt with little signs reading 'Modern Rose Exhibition' and a beautiful Victorian scenic print skirt with carriages and people in fashions of the period. It's a gorgeous print! Besides my 1950s pieces I have a pair of unworn 1920s chestnut-coloured shoes. They are just amazing and were a total bargain for me as I have tiny feet – size 3.

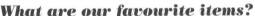

Where do you look to source your vintage fashion items?

I mostly shop online although I love going to the London Vintage Fairs and finding special pieces. I shop a lot on Etsy and eBay and wherever I travel I seek out vintage shops.

What period in fashion history do you find most exciting and why?

I love the 1950s most as it was a really celebratory decade, where fashion seemed to suit everyone and there was a lot of variety. It was all about elegance and looking immaculate. I always loved the film *Grease* from when I first saw it at five years old. I knew even then that I loved the dresses and the colours. I appreciate it more now. I like to read old 1950s clothing catalogues and take inspiration from the styling in them. I adore shows like *Mad Men*; Peggy Olson was a huge inspiration to me in the first few series at the beginning of the 1960s.

What types of materials are particularly easy or hard to find/wear?

I like novelty print rayon; 1940s crepe is getting a lot harder to find and, despite my first purchase, I don't like wearing crimplene.

If someone is thinking about collecting vintage fashion items, what do you suggest they start looking for?

My advice would be to start with a few accessory pieces, find an era that suits you and buy a couple of separates, and shop in places where items from a variety of vintage eras are available.

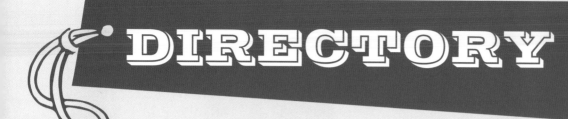

DIRECTORY

Vintage Store	Website
American Classics	www.americanclassicslondon.com/
Bang Bang	bangbangclothingexchange.co.uk/
Blackout II	www.blackout2.com
Collectif	www.collectif.co.uk/
Grays Antique Centre	www.graysantiques.com/index.php
James Smith and Sons	www.james-smith.co.uk/index.cfm
Wow Retro	www.wowretro.co.uk/index.html
Absolute Vintage	www.absolutevintage.co.uk/
Beyond Retro	www.beyondretro.com/en/
Vintage Mode	www.vintagemodes.co.uk/
Decadent Vintage	www.decadentvintage.com/
Fat Faced Cat Vintage	www.fatfacedcat.com/
Glory Days	www.glorydaysvintage.co.uk/
Retro Rehab	www.retro-rehab.co.uk/
The Vintage Wardrobe	www.thevintagewardrobe.com/contact/
Rellik London	www.relliklondon.co.uk/
One Of A Kind	www.oneofakindvintagestore.com/
Paper Dress Vintage	paperdressvintage.co.uk/
Radio Days	www.radiodaysvintage.co.uk/#!
The Looking Glass	stores.ebay.co.uk/The-Looking-Glass-Bridgnorth
Throw Back Vintage	www.facebook.com/throwbackvintage/
Clobber	www.vintageclobber.com/
Ballroom Emporium	www.theballroomemporium.co.uk/
Time After Time	www.stroudvintage.com/
Wolf and Gypsy Vintage	www.wolfandgypsyvintage.co.uk/
Decades Vintage	www.facebook.com/DecadesVintageFashionandTextiles Or www.etsy.com/shop/DecadesUK

Vintage fairs, garage sales, charity shops and thrift shops are all great places to look for vinatge clothes and accessories, but there are many shops that specialize in vintage fashion. The owners are usually very knowledgeable and delighted to help you choose your perfect piece. Below is a small selection of specialst stores.

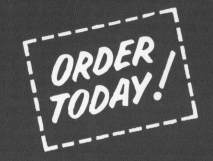

Clothing Type	Eras Covered
Menswear (American)	
Men's, Women's and Accessories	
Men's, Women's and Accessories	20s–80s
Reproduced Womenswear	40s–50s Style
Accessories	–80s
Men's Accessories (Canes, Umbrellas)	
Men's, Women's and Accessories	50s–80s
Vintage & Repro	20s–90s
Men's, Women's and Accessories	
Womenswear and Accessories	
Womenswear and Accessories	
Men's, Women's and Accessories	
Bridal	20s–80s
	50s–90s
	30s–Present
High-End Clothing and Accessories	
Womenswear	20s–80s (20s–90s Accessories)
Men's, Women's and Accessories	
Womenswear	
	20s–80s
Men's, Women's and Accessories	
Men's, Women's and Accessories	
Men's, Women's and Accessories	
Womenswear	
Womenswear	

Cherished	www.cherishedvintage.co.uk/
Deborah Woolf Vintage	www.deborahwoolf.com/
Crazy Man Crazy	www.crazymancrazylondon.co.uk/
Those Were The Days	www.thoseweretthedaysvintage.com/
XANADU VINTAGE	xanaduvintage.com/
Blue 17	www.blue17.co.uk/
Rockit Vintage	www.rokit.co.uk/
Annie's Vintage Costume and Textiles	www.anniesvintageclothing.co.uk/
Retrovert	www.retrovert.co.uk/index.html Or stores.ebay.co.uk/retrovertvintage/
Tara Starlet	www.tarastarlet.com/
Freddies of Pinewood	www.freddiesofpinewood.co.uk/
Vintage Cowboy	www.vintagecowboy.co.uk/
Auntie Aviator	www.facebook.com/Auntie Aviator
Scarlet Rage Vintage	scarletragevintage.com/
Beggars Run	beggarsrun.com/
Froggy Went Courting	www.froggywentcourting.co.uk/
Hopkins Antiques	www.hopkinson21.co.uk/
Madam's Vintage	www.madamsvintage.com/
Alfies Antiques	www.alfiesantiques.com/
Opera Opera	www.operaopera.net/
Rocket Originals	www.rocketoriginals.co.uk/default.asp
Mary Jones Vintage and Glamour	www.maryjonesvintage.com/our-showroom/
Afflecks	www.afflecks.com/
J'Adore Vintage Clothing	www.jadorevintageclothing.co.uk/
Yesterday Society	theyesterdaysociety.co.uk/
Rebecca Jade's Vintage	www.leedsvintage.com/
To Be Worn Again	www.tobewornagain.co.uk/
Mr Ben Retro Clothing	www.mrbenretroclothing.com/index.html
The Glasgow Vintage Co.	glasgowvintage.co.uk/
The Rusty Zip	www.therustyzip.com/
Vintage Vision	www.vintagevision.co.uk/
The Curiosity Shop	curiosityshopbarry.com/retro-shop-south-wales/

Bridal	
Womenswear and Accessories	20s–80s
Men's Clothing	
Men's, Women's and Accessories	
Womenswear	
Men's, Women's and Accessories	50s–80s
Womenswear and Accessories	
Womenswear	20s–80s (Commonly 60s–70s)
Reproduced Womenswear	
Reproduced Menswear and Womenswear	
Cowboy Boots and Leather Accessories	
Vintage Glasses	
Clothing and Accessories	Strong 40s and 50s Stock (and eras between 20s and 70s)
Men's Suits	
Menswear	
Jewellery	
Vintage Glasses	
Jewellery	
Vintage Glasses	
Repro Footwear	40s–50s Casual
Womenswear	
Men's, Women's and Accessories	
Womanswear	20–80s
Menswear and Womenswear	
Womenswear	
Kilo Sale, Menswear and Womenswear	50s–90s
Mix of High-End/ Low-End Menswear, Womenswear and Accessories	30s–90s
Menswear and Womenswear	50s–80s
Menswear and Womenswear	30s–80s
Men's, Womens' and Accessories	50s–90s
Men's, Women's and Accessories	30s–80s

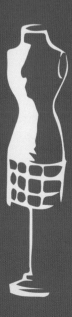

CARING & REPAIRING

If vintage clothing is cared for properly there is no reason why it can't last another 40 plus years. Clothing made from the 1920s to 1950s was made to last. People didn't live in a throwaway society like we do now and didn't have the disposable income to spend on clothing that would only last for one season. Garments were carefully made and looked after to ensure their longevity.

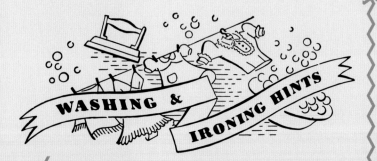

WASHING & IRONING HINTS

CLEAN WITH CARE

Many vintage garments were made before modern washing machines were a household item so they don't come with washing or care instructions. Here are some washing tips for various fabric types. If you're unsure of the fabric take it to a good dry cleaners who can offer advice.

WOOL

Dry clean or hand wash. Using a small amount of soap wash the garment in cool water. Try to avoid rubbing the wool together as it can start to felt. Rinse and place the garment on a towel then roll up and squeeze lightly to remove the excess water. Unroll and leave the clothing to dry out. If there are any wrinkles hang it up in a steamy bathroom.

COTTON

Cotton is a very sturdy fabric so it can be machine washed. Wash on a lingerie/delicates cycle at 30°C (90°F) to make sure the colours stay bright. If you've bought a new item of cotton clothing and you haven't washed it before I would recommend hand washing it. Some dyes used in older garments aren't colourfast so can run. Once dried iron on a cool temperature.

SILK

Dry clean or hand wash in cool water with a gentle detergent. Do not rub the silk against itself as you can damage the fibres. Hang or dry flat. Hang the clothing in a steamy bathroom or, for more stubborn creases, steam or iron at a very low temperature.

ACETATE

Machine or hand wash at a cool temperature. Don't wring the garment out after hand washing. Hang or dry flat (do not tumble dry). Iron while it's still a bit damp at a cool temperature.

POLYESTER

Most items made from polyester can be machine washed and dried as it is a man-made fabric (if unsure do not tumble dry). Polyester can be ironed with a medium-heat iron.

RAYON

Many dresses from the 1940s are made from rayon. They should always be dry cleaned or gently hand washed and ironed at a cool temperature.

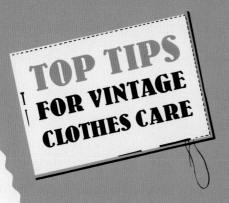

TOP TIPS FOR VINTAGE CLOTHES CARE

• Never hang vintage clothing on metal hangers. Not only are they more likely to snag, they can also alter the shape and even leave rust marks.

• Store clothes out of sunlight. Vintage dyes are often made from natural plants and pigments making them prone to fading. In some cases sunlight can even damage the fibres causing them to perish.

• Keep zips running freely. There's nothing worse than a stiff metal zipper. Simply run a pencil lead or candle up and down the metal teeth to help it run smoothly (it also saves you having to replace it).

• Repair small tears or rips straight away. They will only get bigger if you don't.

• Never iron velvet! I have seen so many beautiful velvet dresses ruined by ironing. It can crush the pile of the fabric. Steam the garment inside out.

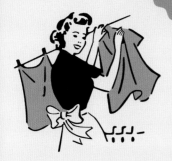

REMOVING STAINS

Before trying to remove a stain always test a spot first to make sure you won't damage the material. When removing the stain, feather the edges to stop a ring from forming.

Place a towel behind the stain to stop the rest of the garment getting wet. Gently blot the stain with a damp clean cloth and warm water. If this doesn't work add a small amount of detergent to the water. Rinse thoroughly with clean warm water and a sponge.

If the stain still persists look out for Vanish soap. You can still buy it in the bar form from some shops. Carefully rub the bar against the stain. Rinse and leave to air dry.

For underarm stains, try dabbing the stain with white vinegar or lemon juice using a clean, lint-free cloth.

For rust stains caused by pins, mix lemon juice with salt and dab on gently.

REMOVING SMELLS

Give the garment a good airing. If that musty smell doesn't disappear, spray it with a mixture of cheap vodka and water. As the liquid evaporates so should the smell. For smaller items, put a small amount of baking soda into a plastic bag with the garment. Shake and leave for a couple of days.

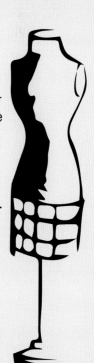

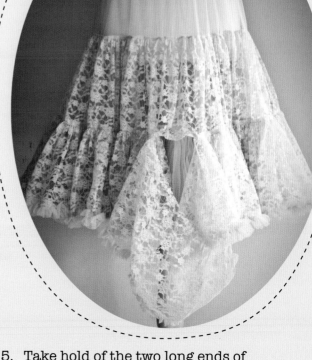

Vintage petticoats are prone to rips and tears. I have repaired this example in a contrasting thread so it's easy to see but you should pick a thread colour as close to the original shade as possible. If you can't find an exact match always go a shade darker. A darker thread will stand out less than a lighter one.

1. Remove any loose threads.

2. Carefully unpick any stitching left from the seam or the gathers.

3. Use the longest stitch length on your sewing machine, and start to sew a line of stitches from one end of the tear 1 cm (½ inch) away from the edge of the tear. Secure the first few stitches by going backwards and forwards a couple of times. When you reach the end of the tear remove the garment from the machine leaving a long thread at both the top and bottom. Do not secure the stitches at the ends.

4. Run another line of stitches parallel to the first line of stitches and the edge of the fabric. Secure the end where you start but not the other end. Remove the garment from the machine leaving a long thread at both the top and bottom.

5. Take hold of the two long ends of thread on top. Move the threads out of the way so they don't get tangled.

6. Gently pull the two threads so the fabric gathers up. Ease the gathers along evenly until the fabric has been pulled up to the correct length (the same length as the layer above).

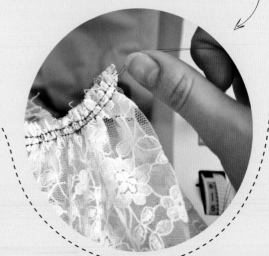

7. Match up the edges of the two layers and secure in place with pins. If you position your pins horizontally you can safely sew over them without the needle breaking. If you are not so confident tack the layers together and remove the pins before moving onto the next step.

8. Change your machine back to a normal stitch length. Starting a couple of inches back from where the hole begins (along the original stitching line). Start sewing. Secure the first few stitches by going backwards and forwards several times.

9. Continue stitching past the hole by a couple of inches along the original seam line. Secure the end by going forwards and backwards a few times. Trim off all of the long threads.

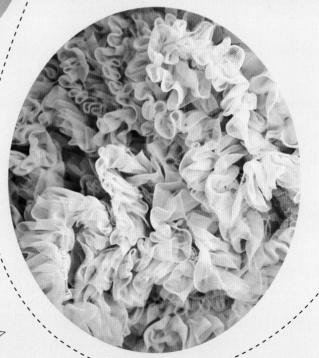

10. If you are worried about the fabric inside fraying and you don't have an overlocker, you can run a zigzag stitch along the raw edge. This will reduce the amount of fraying and also neaten the edge.

11. Turn the garment through to the right side and steam lightly.

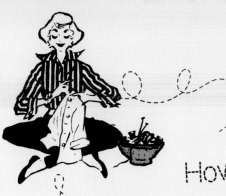

How to let out a dress

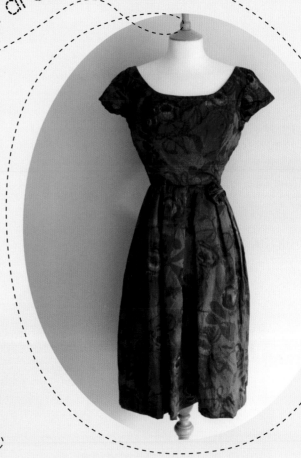

Over the decades body shapes have changed. Many vintage fashions were worn with foundation garments that created a very different shape from those we have today, and generally we're all a lot bigger than we were decades go. There's nothing more frustrating than finding the most perfect dress and discovering that you could do with an extra inch or two. Here's a simple guide to help you gain those vital inches!

Check that there's enough seam before you start unpicking. Also be aware that with some fabrics if you unpick the stitching the fabric may be permanently marked with the original stitching holes.

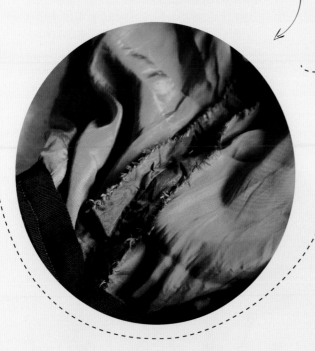

2. Unpick 5cm (2in) of stitching either side of both side seams. Trim any loose threads so that they don't get in the way.

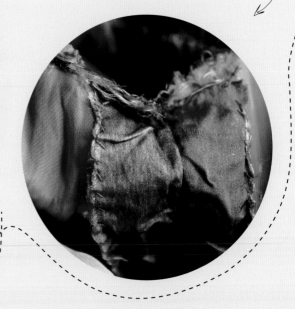

1. Some vintage dresses might have a waist stay (a piece of ribbon with hooks at the waist) inside the garment that helps with zipping the dress up. If you do not have a waist stay continue, if you do, remove it as it will be too small once the alteration is done.

3. If you have a sleeve you will also need to unpick 2.5cm (1in) either side of the underarm seam.

4. If you need to let the dress out as much as possible leave a fairly narrow seam. Don't stitch right on the edge as the fabric might fray and split your side seam. I would suggest a minimum seam allowance of 0.5cm(¼in).

5. With side seams together, pin where you would like your new seam to be. If you have a sleeve you will need to start from the original seam line unless there is enough to let your sleeve out, too.

6. Run a line of tacking stitches along the seam and unpick the original seam. Repeat for the other side.

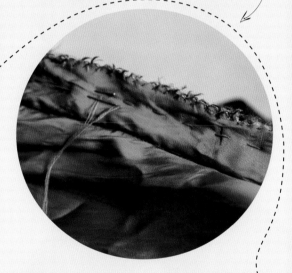

7. On the sewing machine, stitch the new seam line by following the line of tacking. Remember to secure your stitching at both ends by going forwards and backwards several times. Trim loose threads and remove the tacking.

8. Steam out the marks left by the original seam line, placing a cloth over the fabric to avoid damaging it.

9. Pin, tack and re-sew the bodice and sleeve together.

HOW TO LET OUT A SKIRT

You will need to let out the skirt to match the new waist measurement. There are several ways you can do this depending on the style of skirt.

• If your skirt is gathered, simply ease the gathers out. You may have to cut through one of the stitches along the line of gathering to do this.

• If you have a straighter skirt, let out the side seams in the same way that you just let out the bodice seams.

• If you have a pleated skirt, undo a pleat. If the skirt is now too big for the bodice, fold the fabric over slightly to create a smaller pleat. Pin, tack and re-sew the waist together. Use the original stitching line as a guide. Lightly steam/press.

MAKE DO AND MEND

For those wanting to create their own vintage-inspired dresses from vintage fabric think about recycling items such as curtains, sheets and even duvet covers. This is a great way of incorporating vintage fabric into a project and can often be picked up more cheaply than original dressmaking fabrics.

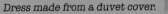

Dress made from a duvet cover.

Tips for vintage fabric shopping

• Check for marks. It can be hard to cut round big marks especially if you're using the width of the fabric for a full skirt.

• Check for holes. The easiest way is to hold up the fabric to the light.

• Make sure that the fabric hasn't perished – if you're using a pair of vintage curtains the light can rot the fabric, causing it to rip.

• Wash the fabric first to make sure that the fabric is pre-shrunk.

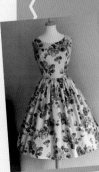

Dress made from original 1950s fabric.

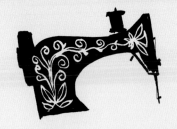

How to replace a zip

Vintage metal zips often break or loose teeth. I think putting a modern zip into a 1950s dress spoils the look of the dress so I try to use vintage zips wherever possible. They're fairly easy to pick up online or in charity shops. I always pick them up whenever I see them especially the longer length ones. The zip on this dress was a modern replacement and had completely split. This is how to replace a lapped zip.

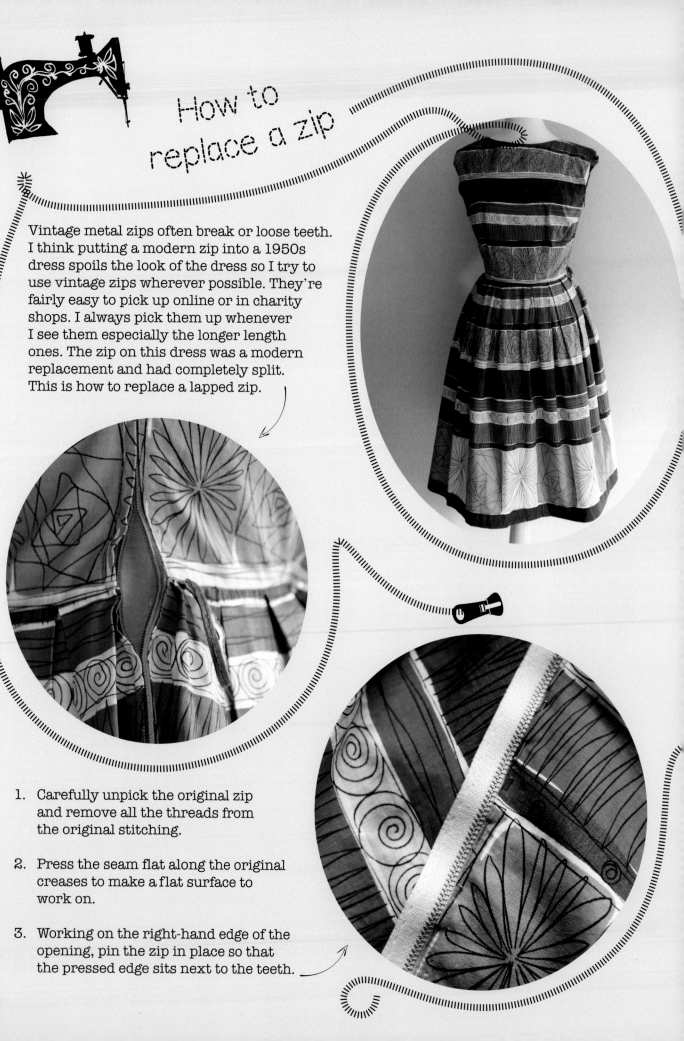

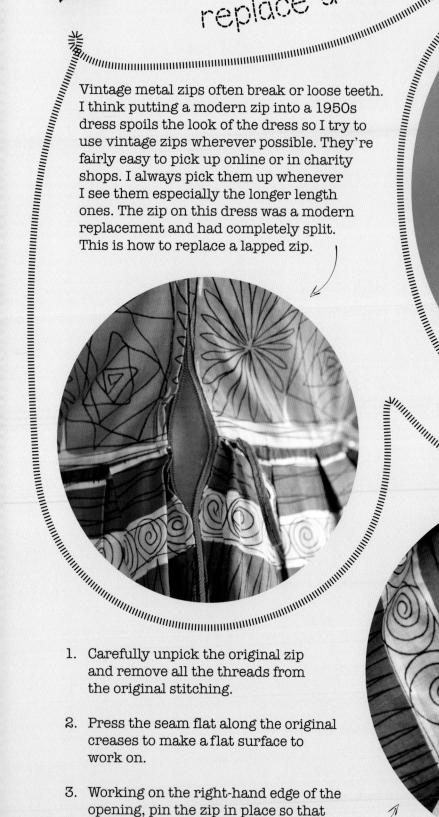

1. Carefully unpick the original zip and remove all the threads from the original stitching.

2. Press the seam flat along the original creases to make a flat surface to work on.

3. Working on the right-hand edge of the opening, pin the zip in place so that the pressed edge sits next to the teeth.

4. Tack the zip in place using a contrasting thread. Remove the pins. Put the zip foot attachment onto your sewing machine.

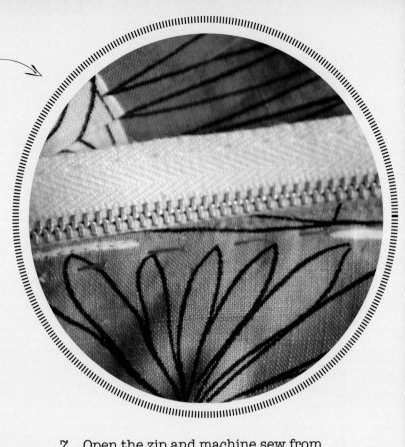

5. Starting at the bottom, top stitch the zip in place. Secure the stitches by going forwards and backwards several times. Remove tacking stitches.

6. Place the left opening edge over the zip so that the zip is hidden and the top stitching is covered. Pin the zip in place making sure that the waist seam and the top of the zip are level. Tack in place approximately 1cm (½in) in from the pressed edge. Remove the pins.

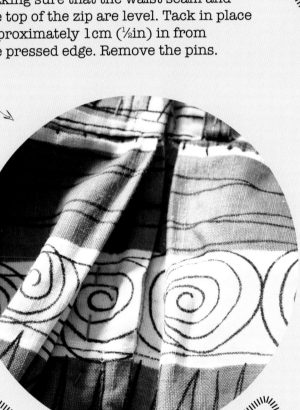

7. Open the zip and machine sew from the top down. As you get closer to the bottom, slide the zip past the needle. If you leave the needle down you will start stitching where you left off.

8. When you get to the bottom leave the needle in and pivot the fabric so that you are stitching across the base of the zip. If you are using a metal zip you could sew across the bottom by winding the needle by hand to ensure that you don't hit the metal and break the needle. Remove all the tacking and press flat.

9. At the top of the zip sew on a hook and eye fastener. Vintage zips tend to slide down and a hook and eye will stop this.

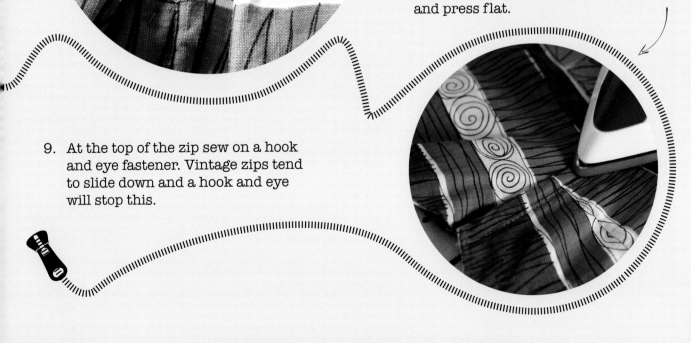

Glossary

acid house A kind of popular synthesized dance music with a fast repetitive beat, popular in the 1980s and associated with taking drugs, such as ecstasy. Acid house parties became popular in the late 1980s and were held in cramped buildings or warehouses. The parties later evolved into raves.

Afghan coat The traditional overcoat of the Afghani tribes, called the posteen or poshteen, which could range from a jacket-to ankle-length, with full or partial sleeves. These coats became very popular In the 1960s and were made from sheepskin or goatskin with the fleece on the inside and the soft suede-like leather on the outside, which was often decorated.

appliqué French for 'applied' or 'laid on'. In its broadest sense, a small piece of ornamental needlework sewn or stuck on to another larger surface.

Armani, Giorgio (1934–) Italian fashion designer, particularly noted for his menswear. His popularity increased in the 1980s when his men's 'power suits' were featured in the American television series *Miami Vice* and in Hollywood films, and wearing Armani became a symbol of success for many businessmen. He is known today for his clean, tailored lines and launched his first haute couture line in 2005. Armani has now expanded his business to include hotels.

Art Deco A style of art, decoration and architectural design that first appeared in France after World War I and which flourished internationally in the 1920s and 1930s. It is recognized by strong lines, geometric motifs, bold colours and the use of new materials, such as plastic .

Art Nouveau A style of decorative art, architecture, and design that was prominent in western Europe and the USA from about 1890 until World War I. Characterized by intricate linear designs and flowing curves based on natural forms. The style went out of fashion after it gave way to Art Deco in the 1920s.

asymmetric shaping The absence of, or a violation of, symmetry, where there is no balance on both sides of a central line. In design or clothes, this means that one side is not the same as the other or that one limb (shoulder/arm or knee/leg) is given greater exposure.

atelier French for a workshop or studio, especially one used by a designer where designs are created and made up.

'baby boom' Following the end of World War II there was a rapid increase in the birth rate, which is often referred to as a 'baby boom'. People born between the years 1946 and 1964 are known as 'baby boomers'.

bakelite An early type of brittle plastic used mainly for its electrical nonconductivity and heat resistant properties, for example in radio and telephone casings and in products ranging from kitchenware to jewellery, to firearms and children's toys. The 'retro' appeal of old Bakelite products has made them collectible.

Bargello needlework A type of needlepoint embroidery consisting of upright flat stitches laid in a mathematical pattern that create a variety of zigzag designs and motifs.

Beat Generation American writer Jack Kerouac introduced the phrase 'Beat Generation' in 1948, generalizing from his social circle to characterize the underground, anti-conformist youth gathering in New York at that time.

beatniks A young person in 1950s to early 1960s associated with the Beat Generation, the literary movement of the 1950s. One who rejects conventional society and chooses to express themselves through art and adopting a style of dress that included dark glasses, black trousers, black polo neck jumpers and black berets.

Bellville, Sassoon Fashion house founded by Belinda Bellville in 1953.

bespoke trousers Trousers (or any items) that are specially commissioned to a particular specification or made to order. They may be altered or tailored to the customer's taste or the usage of an individual purchaser.

birdcage lace Broadly woven, delicate lace resembling a birdcage that was worn as a veil across the face. It was a popular addition to women's hats in the 1940s.

bishop sleeve A long sleeve, fuller at the bottom than the top, and gathered into a cuff at the wrist. A style adapted from that worn by some church bishops.

black market When goods or services are traded illegally. 'Black' market might have had started with fire damaged goods – or rather goods that were supposed to have been lost in a fire, but were really sold through 'unconventional' outlets.

blackout cloth Black cotton cloth that stopped the light from rooms showing outside at night during World War II. The idea was to stop lights from towns guiding enemy planes to drop bombs on buildings.

body-con Short for body-conscious; a style of very tight-fitting clothing that emphasizes the contours of the body.

Bodymap An influential British fashion label of the 1980s, renowned for its layered and innovatively structured and unstructured shapes, distinctive prints and groundbreaking fashion shows. The clothes were designed for the young, avant garde and daring, and produced mainly in black, white and cream.

BoHo chic A style of fashion drawing on various bohemian and hippie influences.

'Bold Look' The men's version of Dior's 'New Look' from 1947 and 1948 featuring looser, baggier suits often with a wide pin stripe pattern and brightly coloured ties with bold checks or stripes.

box pleats Formed when two equal folds of fabric are folded away from each other in opposite directions; they usually spring out from the waistline.

'Bright Young Things' or 'Bright Young People' Nickname for a group of fashionable young aristocrats and socialites noted for their outrageous behaviour.

Brit Pop A subgenre of rock and pop music that emerged from the British independent music scene of the early 1990s. Influenced by British pop music of the 1960s, especially music by the Beatles, and indie rock from the 1980s. It was seen as a reaction against American grunge music.

brogue A style of man's low-heeled shoe or boot traditionally with multiple-piece leather uppers with decorative perforations ('broguing') and serration along the visible edges.

Brooks, Louise (1906–1985) An American dancer and actress, noted for popularizing the bobbed haircut. She made her film debut in 1925, and perhaps her most memorable role was as the amoral, self-destructive temptress Lulu in *Pandora's Box*.

buffalo A Caribbean expression to describe people who are rude boys or rebels. Not necessarily tough, but hard style taken from the street – a functional and stylish look; non-fashion with a hard attitude'.

Capri pants Tight fitting, mid-calf trousers worn by women, especially in the United States, Europe, Latin America and Asia. Their name derives from the Italian island of Capri where the trousers first became popular in the late 1950s.

Cardin, Pierre (1922–) Italian-born French designer known for his geometric, avant-garde style and his Space Age designs. In the 1960s Cardin showcased innovation in men's fashions with the so-called Nehru Jacket and went on to introduce neck scarves in place of ties, and turtlenecks instead of button-down shirts. During the early 1960s, Cardin was a pioneer in designing clothing conspicuously adorned with his company's logo. This trend was picked up by many other designers from the 1970s.

Cartier Internationally recognized high end jewellery brand founded in 1847 by Louis-Françoise Cartier.

Central Saint Martins (or CSM) A public art school in London formed in1989 from the merger of St Martin's School of Art and the Central School of Arts & Crafts. In 1999 it was joined by the Drama Centre London, which introduced acting and directing to the art and design environment.

Chanel, Coco (1883–1971) Gabrielle Bonheur 'Coco' Chanel a French fashion designer who founded the Chanel brand. She is credited with liberating women from the constraints of the 'corseted silhouette' by creating a relaxed, comfortable style for women with collarless cardigan jackets, boxy cardigan suits and her signature little black dress. Chanel's world famous fragrance, No.5, was launched in 1922.

cheongsam A long, straight, body-hugging dress with a high collar and slit skirt, worn traditionally by Chinese and Indonesian women.

chignon A popular hairstyle comprising a knot or coil of hair arranged at the back of the neck. The word "chignon" comes from the French phrase 'chignon du cou', which means bun at the nape of the neck.

Classic shirt Boxy shape, generously cut across the shoulders, chest, waist and hips, with long tails.

cloche hat A fitted, bell-shaped hat for women invented in 1908 by milliner Caroline Reboux. Derived from *cloche*, the French word for 'bell'.

clothing coupon allowance In 1941, the British government introduced clothes rationing to ensure an equal distribution of clothing. Each person was issued with a maximum of just 66 clothing coupons per year (this was reduced to 40 coupons in 1943). This equated to one outfit a year

Cool Britannia A phrase used to describe a period of increased pride in the culture of Britain throughout most of the 1990s inspired by 1960s pop culture. It was used to promote Britain to a world audience.

couturier French for dressmaker. A top international fashion designer who manufactures and sells clothes that have been tailored to a client's specific requirements and measurements.

Cox, Patrick (1963–) Canadian-British fashion designer, specializing in shoes, leather goods and accessories. In the 1990, Cox designed the Wannabe shoe that was so successful that a queue of 200 people formed outside his shop and the design sold over 100,000 pairs a season.

crepe de chine A soft, fine silk, wool or synthetic fibre fabric with a distinctively crisp, crimped appearance.

crew cut A very short haircut for men and boys. The hair on the sides and back of the head is short while the top is just slightly longer, like the bristles on a brush. The hairstyle was popular with college students in the United States (especially Ivy League rowers) in the 1920s and 1930s, and with American GIs in World War II.

cubism An early twentieth century style and art movement that emphasized the geometrical depiction of natural forms. Pablo Picasso was one of the leading cubists.

cummerbund A wide waist sash, usually pleated, worn with single-breasted dinner jackets or tuxedos.

décolletage The area that covers a woman's chest from the neckline down to the cleavage; a low neckline on a woman's dress or top.

denier The unit of weight (or thickness) by which the fineness of silk, rayon or nylon hosiery yarn is measured. Generally, the lower the denier, the sheerer the appearance.

Dior, Christian (1905–1957) In 1947, aged 42 years, Dior presented his first collection in Paris, which became known as the 'New Look'.

dolman sleeves (from Turkish dolaman robe) Originally referred to a long, loose garment with narrow sleeves and an opening at the front worn by Turks. A dolman sleeve is set into a very low armhole and gathered at the wrist; it is cut in one piece with the body of the garment.

duchesse satin A soft, shiny, heavy and luxurious fabric often used for couture wedding gowns and evening wear.

enamelling The technique of using heat to fuse powdered glass to a metal surface to add decoration or colour.

Eton crop A very short hairstyle adopted by women in the 1920s, named for the style worn by boys attending Eton public school.

Fish, Michael (Mr Fish) (1940–) Started his fashion career by working for a couple of renowned fashion houses and shirt makers in London in the 50s and early 60s until he decided to open his own shop MR FISH in London in 1966. Fish is regarded as the inventor of kipper ties, a trendsetter for the polo neck sweater look and as one of the protagonists of the so-called *Peacock Revolution*, which marked the change to more colourful designs for men's clothing.

flapper A name given to the new 'breed' of young western women in the 1920s who wore short skirts, bobbed their hair, listened to jazz and flaunted their disdain for what was then considered acceptable behaviour.

Fratini, Gina (1931–) Established her own fashion house in the 1960s in London and became one of the top British fashion designers of the early 1970s. Known for her romantic designs, incorporating ruffles, laces and lavish embroidery into multi-layered, soft dresses with delicate prints.

French or ticket pockets Small third pockets on jackets and blazers. Traditionally, these were a distinctly British detail, but today they often feature on pieces from America, Italy and many other. countries

von Fürstenberg, Diane (1946–) Formerly Princess Diane of Fürstenberg, a Belgian-born American fashion designer and creator of the iconic knitted jersey wrap dress that went on sale in 1974.

garçonne French equivalent of the British flapper – a young woman who rebelled against conventional ideas of ladylike behaviour and who adopted a boyish look.

Givenchy, Hubert de (1927–) French designer who founded the House of Givenchy in 1952. Givenchy's debut Separates collection included light floor-length skirts that were interchangeable with blouses. In 1954, he became the first couturier to present a luxury ready-to-wear line. His design philosophy was simplicity and this was further established in 1957 with one of his most influential designs, the revolutionary sack dress. He said, "The dress must follow the body of the woman, not the body following the shape of the dress."

godet A triangular piece of material inserted in a dress, shirt, or glove to make it flared or for ornamentation.

Great Depression The long, severe worldwide financial and industrial slump of 1929 and for most of the 1930s.

grunge A subculture of alternative rock that emerged during the mid 1980s in the US state of Washington, particularly in Seattle. It was characterized by a harsh, loud guitar sound and lazy vocal style. Fashion associated with grunge included loose, layered clothing and ripped jeans.

Gucci, Guccio (1881–1953) Opened his own leather goods store in his native Florence in 1921. With his sons, Gucci expanded the company to feature more shops that sold finely crafted accessories including handbags, shoes, silks and knitwear and, later, watches.

'Halston', Roy Halston Frawick (1932–1990) American fashion designer known as Halston, synonymous with the disco scene of the 1970s.

hand-span belt (also called a waist cincher) A small corset usually worn over a girdle to make the wearer's waist smaller. It became the quintessential undergarment of Dior's New Look in the late 1940s.

harem pants Full, loose-fitting trousers made of soft material that is gathered in closely at the ankle. They were introduced to western fashion by couturier Paul Poiret, around 1910 inspired by Middle East styles and by şalvar (Turkish trousers).

haute couture French for 'high sewing', 'high dressmaking' or 'high fashion'. The term refers to the exclusive, made to measure clothes produced by leading fashion houses.

hourglass silhouette The hourglass corset was worn to produce a silhouette resembling the hourglass shape: wide bottom, narrow waist (wasp waist), wide top.

'Ivy League' college One of a group eight old, highly distinguished universities or colleges in the northeastern United States, so-called because their buildings invariably had ivy covered walls.

Juliet cap A small open-work crocheted or mesh cap, often decorated with pearls, beads or jewels, mainly worn with evening gowns or as bridal wear. The cap is named after the heroine of Shakespeare's *Romeo and Juliet*.

jump suit Originally a one-piece garment worn by skydivers, the jump suit became a staple of 1970s and 1980s fashion.

Kabuki theatre Kabuki is a classical Japanese dance-drama known for the stylization of its acting, movement and songs, and the elaborate costumes and make-up worn by some of its performers.

Klein, Calvin (1942–) His first designs focused on women's coats. In the 1970s, he launched the first range of designer jeans. In addition to clothing for men and women, Klein has also given his name to a range of perfumes, cosmetics, watches and jewellery.

Lacroix, Christian (1951–) Born in France, Lacroix launched his own haute couture house in 1987 and helped to define the look of the 1980s, combining bright colours and extravagant detail, such as ornamental embroidery with contemporary shapes. He has diversified his design interest into jeans, perfume, children's wear, lingerie, mens wear couture, ready-to-wear and homeware.

Lauren, Ralph (1939–) American fashion designer best known for his sportswear line Polo, which now includes clothing for men, women and children, fragrances, home furnishings and luxury clothing.

Laurent, Yves Saint (1935–2008) Born in Algeria, Saint Laurent moved to Paris where his designs quickly gained notice and he started work under the guidance of designer Christian Dior. In 1961 he produced designs such as blazers and the classic tuxedo suit for women, Le Smoking suit (1966), and signature pieces included the sheer blouse and the jumpsuit. Saint Laurent said, "Chanel freed women, and I empowered them."

layered shag A hairstyle which is shorter in the front and longer in the back with many layers to give a soft, messy look.

leg-of-mutton sleeve (also the gigot sleeve and leg of lamb sleeve) Acquired its name because of its unusual shape; voluminous at the top and close-fitting on the forearm and wrist. The sleeve's shape resembled a lamb shank.

leitmotif A recurrent theme associated with a particular person, situation or idea.

loafers (slip-ons) Casual, low heeled step-in shoes with an upper resembling a moccasin.

loons Trousers made from cotton, velvet or corduroy. So-called because they hugged the leg to the knee and then 'ballooned' out into a wide flare.

marcasite A semi-precious stone with a bronze-yellow colour.

metal segs or blakeys Metal studs or plates fixed to the toe, sole or heel of shoes for protection and to avoid excessive wear.

Miyake, Issey (1938–) Japanese fashion designer known for his technology-driven clothing, exhibitions and fragrances.

mods (or modernists) Great rivals of the rockers, the mods rode decorated scooters, liked soul, blues and ska music, and wore suits and parka jackets. The mod subculture has its roots in a small group of London-based stylish young men in the late 1950s who were termed modernists because they listened to modern jazz.

moire A fabric with a wavy (watered) appearance produced mainly from silk, but can also be made from wool, cotton and rayon.

Muir, Jean (1928–1995) British dressmaker who made clothes that were both radical and classical, breaking the barrier between couture and ready-to-wear. Muir was self-taught and made her name in the 1960s by producing exquisitely tailored, timeless, feminine designs.

musquash A medium-sized semi-aquatic rodent native to North America also known as the muskrat.

New Romantics A style of music and fashion popular in Britain in the early 1980s in which both men and women wore make-up and dressed in flamboyant clothes. The movement is often seen as a direct reaction to the British punk scene of the 1970s.

notch lapels (step lapels or step collar) The most common style of lapel found on single-breasted suit jackets, blazers and sports jackets. The lapels are sewn to the collar at an angle creating a step effect.

Nutter, Tommy (1943–1992) A British tailor, famous for reinventing the Savile Row suit in the 1960s. Nutter combined traditional tailoring skills with innovative design. In the 1980s, he described his suits as a "…cross between the big-shouldered *Miami Vice* look and the authentic Savile Row."

Op art (or Optical art) A style of abstract visual art that used optical effects and illusions to fool the eye of the viewer. The abstract patterns employed were often in black and white for maximum contrast. The movement saw its greatest success in the mid 1960s.

Oxford bags Loose-fitting, trousers with wide baggy legs named for their popularity with members of the University of Oxford, especially undergraduates, from the 1920s to around the 1950s.

Paletot cut (or the pilot coat or paleot) A man's semi-fitted to fitted usually double-breasted top coat with peaked lapels, usually made of a dark, plain fabric.

parachute pants A style of trousers characterized by the use of nylon, especially ripstop nylon (extra strong and reinforced nylon), the material used to make parachutes. Originally created for break dancers, the trousers were shiny and tight-fitting with several decorative pockets and zips .

pea coat (or pea jacket, pilot jacket) An coat, generally double-breasted and made of a navy-coloured heavy wool, originally worn by sailors of European and later American navies.

peaked lapel Lapel edges that point upwards and towards the shoulder. Traditionally these lapels were seen on formal garments, such as tailcoats, but are nearly always seen of double-breasted jackets or coats.

percale A closely woven, fine, cotton fabric used for sheets and clothing.

PETA (People for the Ethical Treatment of Animals) An American animal rights organization based in Norfolk, Virginia, founded in 1980.

Petri, Ray (1948 – 1989) Fashion deisgner and stylist and creator of the fashion house, Buffalo.

piqué appliqué A strongly ribbed or raised pattern that is used to decorate an aspect of a garment or product.

Plus fours Baggy knickerbockers that reach 10 cm (4 in) below the knee, and are 10cm longer than traditional knickerbockers, hence their name. Plus fours were formerly worn by men for hunting and golf.

Poiret, Paul (1879–1944) A leading French fashion designer during the first two decades of the 20th century. Poiret produced many new, innovative designs, which led to the abandonment of the 's' bend corset in favour of the straight, upright silhouette in dresses. He introduced the hobble skirt, harem pants and cocoon and kimono coats. He used vivid colours and oriental-inspired designs and is credited for pioneering both boutique and ready-to-wear ranges. Poiret was the first designer to develop a fragrance line.

pop art An art movement that emerged in the mid-1950s and flourished in the 1960s in Britain and the United States (especially New York City). It drew inspiration from sources in popular and commercial culture, such as advertising and comic books. Key artists include Andy Warhol, Roy Lichtenstein, Peter Blake and David Hockney.

'preppy look' Preppy or prep (abbreviations of the word preparatory) refer to a subculture in the United States associated with the old northeastern Ivy League universities or preparatory academies. The terms are used to denote a person who wears a style of clothing associated with these institutions eg, a monogrammed blazer or jumper with the initial letter of your college was a classic preppy outfit.

psychedelic Relating to drugs, especially LSD, that produce hallucinations, distortions of perception and altered states of awareness. Psychedelic clothing included intense vivid colour and swirling abstract patterns.

Pucci, Emilio (1914 – 1992) Italian fashion designer and politician. He and his eponymous company are synonymous with geometric prints in a kaleidoscope of colours. His collections included designs made from stretch silk and cotton jersey and included elegant styles which took women from day to evening and from jets to cocktail parties, heralding the concept of designer ready-to wear.

punk First emerged in London in the mid 1970s. An anarchic aggressive anti-establishment, anti-fashion subculture that became popular with the success of Vivienne Westwood and partner Malcolm McLaren.

pyrite (also called fool's gold) A shiny yellow metallic mineral used to make marcasite jewellery, often set in silver.

Quant, Mary Dame (1934 –) British designer and fashion icon, Mary Quant opened a boutique in London in 1955 when "fashion wasn't designed for young people" introducing the 'mod era' and the 'Chelsea look'. Quant's designs were made up of simple shapes combined with strong colours. In 1963 she opened a second shop and later launched the Ginger Group, a line of lower priced designs to appeal to an even wider clientele. In the late 1960s she went on to popularize hot pants.

Rabanne, Paco Francisco (1934–) 'Paco' Rabaneda y Cuervo, French fashion designer of Spanish origin. In 1965 he presented his first collection of 12 contemporary dresses, which he called 'the Unwearables'. In 1966 Rabanne produced dresses made of small plastic tiles linked together by chains, which stole the show in Paris. He was also known as a costume designer for the cinema, theatre and ballet, and was the first to use black girls as models, which was considered quite outrageous at the time.

rave scene Psychedelic and electronic dance music, most notably acid house music and techno, played in clubs, warehouses and free-parties first in Manchester in the mid 1980s and later London. The first warehouse parties in Manchester were organized by the rock group Stone Roses in 1985, when to get around the licensing laws they would play a gig and book a line-up of DJs under the disused arches of Piccadilly train station.

reefer The traditional term for short, heavy, close-fitting double-breasted woollen jacket traditionally worn by sailors.

Rhodes, Zandra Dame (1940–) One of the new wave of British designers who put London at the forefront of the international fashion scene in the 1970s. With her love of printed textile design, Rhodes produced dresses from her own fabrics with bold prints, feminine patterns and theatrical use of colour. She has extended her range of designs from dresses to include jewellery, wrapping paper, china and make-up, and in 2003 set up the Fashion and Textile Museum in London.

rockers Members of a biker subculture originating in Britain that evolved out of the Teddy Boys during the 1950s. Rockers' 'uniform' comprised a heavy black leather jacket, which was often decorated, denim jeans and black leather with white socks rolled over the tops of the boots. Their focus was centred on motorcycles and rock and roll music.

'rude boy' style A subculture that arose from the poorer sections of Kingston, Jamaica, and was associated with violent discontented youths who favoured sharp suits, thin ties and pork pie or trilby hats.

Schiaparelli, Elsa (1890–1973) Italian-born French couturière best known for the bold and brazen originality of her work. She loved to flout convention in pursuit of a more idiosyncratic style and enlisted the talents of many artisans and artists, particularly those associated with the Surrealist movement. Schiaparelli's designs incorporated themes inspired by current events, erotic fantasy, traditional and avant-garde art and her own psyche, using experimental fabrics with pronounced textures, bold prints and unorthodox imagery and colours.

sheath dress A fairly plain, straight, tight-fitting dress.

Shrimpton, Jean (1942–) Top model of the 1960s discovered by photographer David Bailey.

ska music A genre originating in Jamaica in the late 1950s and the precursor to rocksteady and reggae. Ska is a fusion of American jazz, African and Calypso rhythms with rhythm and blues.

'slave bangles' Bangles or bracelets worn above the elbow.

Smith, Paul Sir (1946–) British men's fashion designer.. He has described his designs as "… well-made, good quality, simple cut, interesting fabric, easy to wear" and often adds a splash of vibrant colour, a floral print or his signature multi-coloured stripes. Today, Smith produces collections for both men and women.

smock dress (or smock) Traditionally a loose fitting, outer shirt-like garment made of heavy linen or wool and gathered onto a yoke and decorated with smocking. It was worn by rural workers, such as shepherds. In the 1960s, a smock was a dress or blouse gathered at the top and with a loose fitting lower part.

Spandex (an anagram of 'expands') A type of polyurethane fabric popular for its exceptional elasticity, also known as Lycra. It is often used in sportswear.

Spanx Body-shaping undergarments which are intended to give the wearer a slim and smooth appearance.

spats Short for spatterdashes, or spatter guards), type of cloth gaiter worn over outdoor shoes, they cover the instep and usually fasten under the foot with a strap. White spats worn over polished black shoes, together with a top hat and cane, were often worn in the late 19th and early 20th century by wealthy men.

spectator shoe Low-heeled, oxford, semi-brogue or full-brogue shoe constructed from two contrasting colours, typically having the toe and heel cap and sometimes the lace panels in a darker colour from the main body of the shoe.

spiv A type of petty criminal, usually a flashy dresser, who deals in illicit, typically black market goods.

Studio 54 An extremely popular New York nightclub frequented by the rich and famous from 1977 to 1979 located at 254 West 54th Street in Manhattan.

surrealism A 20th century avant-garde movement in art and literature which sought to release the creative potential of the unconscious mind – it aimed at expressing imaginative dreams and visions free from conscious rational control.

'Swinging London' A term coined by *Time* magazine in April 1966. This was a catch-all phrase applied to the fashion and cultural scene that flourished in London in the 1960s. It emphasized the young, the new and the modern during a period of optimism and hedonism, and a cultural revolution.

tank top A close-fitting sleeveless top usually knitted and worn over a shirt or blouse. The term derived from its resemblance to a tank suit, a style of one-piece women's swimsuit of the 1920s worn in tanks or swimming pools.

tea dress (or tea gown) A semi-formal dress made of fine material, especially one styled with soft, flowing lines, worn for afternoon social occasions.

Teddy Boys (also known as Teds) A British subculture started in the 1950s, typified by young men wearing clothes that were partly

inspired by the styles worn by dandies in the Edwardian period. Originally known as Cosh Boys, the name Teddy Boy was coined when a 1953 *Daily Express* newspaper headline shortened Edwardian to Teddy.

tonneau-shaped watches A watch case or dial resembling a barrel in profile.

'Twiggy' (Lesley Hornby) (1949–) Model, actress and singer known for her thin build (hence her nickname) and her androgynous look.

Ulster overcoat Originally a Victorian daytime overcoat with a cape and sleeves, the Ulster has evolved into a long, heavy overcoat, usually double-breasted, and made from Donegal tweed. It is so-called because it was originally produced in Northern Ireland.

utilitari Designed to be useful or practical rather than attractive.

Valentino (Valentino Garavani) (1932–) Italian fashion designer best known as Valentino created some of the world's most elegant evening wear and classic designs. His international debut took place in 1962 in Florence and was a great success. After this breakthrough show Valentino became the designer favoured by royalty, film stars and socialites. He drew particular praise for his full-length skirts (which flew in the face of the new wave of minis), his signature 'Valentino red' and his love for the simple contrast of black and white. Valentino delivered his last women's ready-to-wear show in Paris in 2008 before retiring.

Victorian dress shirt A shirt with a stylish high stand collar, worn for formal evening wear.

Wall Street Crash When, in 1929, the value of shares on the Wall Street Stock Exchange in New York fell so low that many people lost all their money. This led to the Great Depression of the 1930s.

Westward, Vivienne Dame (1941–) British fashion designer largely responsible for bringing modern punk and new wave fashions into the mainstream.

wide boys (synonymous with spivs) Men involved in wheeling and dealing, usually involving petty crimes.

Yuppies Short for 'young urban professional' or 'young upwardly-mobile professional', used to describe a young, ambitious, college-educated adult who has a high-paid job and an affluent lifestyle.

zoot suit An exaggerated dress style, characterized by a long loose jacket with wide lapels, padded shoulders and high-waisted, tapering trousers, often worn with braces, a long watch chain and a large-brimmed fedora-style hat. They were generally worn by young men of African-American, and Mexican-American descent and also by white working-class men.

About the Authors

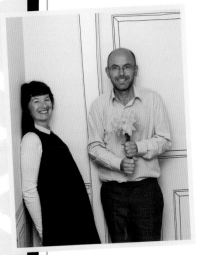

Wayne Hemingway MBE, and his wife Gerardine, have been involved with the fashion business since they were teenagers. Famously emptying their wardrobes onto Camden Market at the turn of the 80s, Wayne and Gerardine went on to create the iconic fashion label, Red or Dead, when they were 20 and 19 respectively, and sold it in the late 90s. Since then they have established a hugely successful multi-disciplinary design company, HemingwayDesign, specializing in homewares and exhibitions. Wayne's passion for vintage inspired him to set up the Vintage Festival and Classic Car Boot Sale events in the UK in 2007 that attract hundreds of thousands of aficionados from around the world every year. The Hemingways also co-own a quirky museum, The Land of Lost Content, and from this they have created an impressive private image library. The Land of Lost Content is the inspiration for *The Vintage Fashion Bible*, and the majority of images in the book come from this source.

Contributors

Get the Look with Hannah/Ask the Expert: Make-up

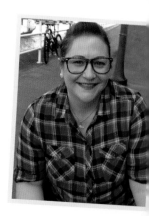

Hannah Wing started her make-up business in 2007 and was soon approached to become the senior make-up artist for a leading airbrush cosmetic brand, working on film and television programmes as well as catwalks and magazines features. Since then Hannah has continued to work on a wide variety of projects and gone on to train industry professionals as well as lecturing in media hair and make-up at colleges around the UK. Hannah's love of vintage and flair for styling saw her launch her own company, Petite Vintage Boudoir in 2015, which specializes in selling original vintage items and offers a personal vintage shopper and styling service www.petitevintageboudoir.co.uk. Her book, *The Vintage Beauty Parlor*, was published in 2013. Visit Hannah at www.bellusfemina.co.uk

Caring & Repairing

Emma Golding started her vintage reproduction clothing company Oh Sew Vintage when she was 18. All of Emma's dresses are made from original vintage patterns using high quality fabrics. She attends vintage fairs around the country and is based at No38 Vintage Emporium in Newport Pagnal and the Hertfordshire Craft Collective in Radlett, Hertfordshire. Emma also offers vintage sewing classes.

Ask the Expert: Collecting

Holly Foster is a 22-year-old office worker who wears vintage clothes almost every day. In addition to her day job, Holly both acts and sings, writes historical fiction and loves swing dances. She has been a collector of vintage fashion for the last few years.

Ask the Expert: Buttons

Martyn Firth's mother, Toni, started the Button Queen empire in the 1950s and Martyn now runs it with his wife, Isabel. The shop is located in central London. www.thebuttonqueen.co.uk

Ask the Expert: Hats

Quonah Foster was initially inspired to take up millinery following a course with couture milliner, Prudence, and after further studies with leading international milliner, Noel Stewart, at Kensington and Chelsea College, she set up MaidenFound Millinery in 2010 based in London, where she lives with her cat, Paisley. She creates affordable bespoke headpieces using traditional millinery techniques and materials, specializing in vintage-inspired headwear for every occasion and outfit. Quonah has customers from all over the UK and abroad, and likes the process of creating a bespoke headpiece to be a creative and enjoyable experience for the customer. Contact her at www.maidenfound.com

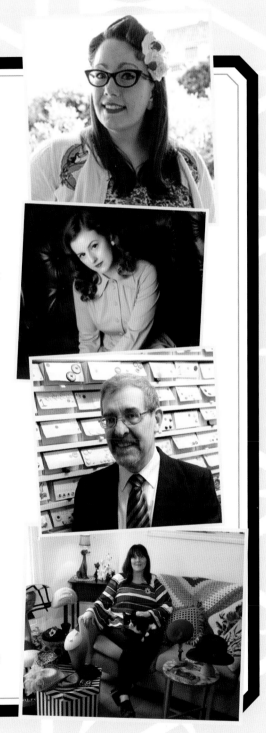

Picture Credits

Index

1920s 12, 14–31, 33, 52, 104
1930s 34–51, 52, 105
1940s 53, 54–77, 106, 136, 201
1950s 33, 53, 78–101, 107, 201
1960s 53, 112–31, 189
1970s 53, 109, 134–59, 189
1980s 53, 110, 160–183
1990s 110, 184–93

accessories 28–9, 48–50, 74–5, 98–100, 128–9, 156–7, 180–1
acetate 206
Adidas 126, 127, 154, 177, 179
adjusting garments 210–11
animal prints 173
Armani, Giorgio 144
art, and fashion 116
Ashley, Laura 115

badges 156
bags 49, 50
  Chanel flap 181
  clutch 29, 31, 49, 76
  granny 76
  'man' 75
  shoulder 157
  sports 127
bandeau 31
basketball chic 178
Beatlemania 113, 121, 125
Beatniks 113, 119, 120
'beau, return of the' 86

belts 141
  cage 67
bias cut 40
Biba 117
'big look' ('droop look') 140, 165
bikinis 96
Blitz club, The 175
blouses 59
body tights 149
boho chic 137, 158
Bolan, Marc 151
'Bold Look' 62, 68
bondage 138
boob tubes 146
boots 71, 125
  Chelsea 125
  Dr Martens 176
  knee highs 177
Bowie, David 9, 137
bowling chic 127
bows 141
boxing chic 126
Boy George 167, 175, 181
braces 28, 183
Braemer 46
bras 196
  cone (bullet) 82
'Bright Young Things' 12, 15
Brit Pop 186
buttons 52–3
buying vintage 13, 196–205, 211

canes 39
capes 138
cardigans 85, 145

Cardin, Pierre 121
caring for garments 206–13
Chanel 17, 20, 41, 53, 180–1
Chanel, Coco 15, 16, 26, 31, 49
charity shops 62, 136
Charlie's Angels 158
chokers 191
cleaning garments 206–7
coats 42–3
  duffle 87
  Mackintoshes 38
  maxi 115
  morning 43
  swing 83
  tailcoats 22, 23, 42, 68
  top 92
  see also jackets
collars 28, 39, 43, 150–1
compacts 133
'Cool Britannia' 186
cotton 206
cravats 108–10, 129
cricket wear 27
crimping 183
crochet 138
cummerbunds 93
cycling chic 27

dance fashions 21, 57, 72, 146, 149–50, 161, 164, 170, 174–5, 178–9, 186–7
day wear
  men's 18–19, 38–9, 60–3, 84–7, 118–21, 142–5, 169–71

women's 16–17, 36–7, 56–9, 80–3, 114–17, 136–9, 162–5
de Lennart, Sonja 80
décolletage 64, 67, 90, 99
denim 138, 141, 143, 163, 188
Diana, Princess of Wales 172
Dior, Christian 12, 33, 53, 94, 156, 180
  New Look 64, 66, 79, 91
disco 146, 149, 150, 155, 158, 164
Dr Martens 176
drapes, shoulder 29, 37
dresses 40–1
  ball gowns 91
  cocktail 88, 172
  halter-neck 90
  house 81
  letting out 210–11
  paper 116
  V-neck 90
  wedding 104–11
  wrap 149
dungarees 57, 144
Dynasty (TV series) 173

Eastern styles 123
Edward VIII 19, 35, 42–3
embellishments 33, 66, 89, 122
equestrian wear 97
evening wear
  men's 22–3, 42–3, 68–9, 92–3, 150–1, 174–5
  women's 20–1, 40–1,

64–7, 88–91, 122–3, 146–9, 172–3
eyeliner 100

facial hair 51, 195
fake labels 198
family outfits 144
Far Eastern styles 146
Ferragamo, Salvatore 44, 71
Fila 179
Fish, Michael 118, 151
'fitness' fashion 161, 185
flapper girls 16, 31
floral prints 115, 187
football fashion 127
Foster, Holly 200–1
Foster, Quonah 32–3
fragrance 31, 51, 62, 129, 158, 199
fur 29, 37, 173
  faux 91, 142
future vintage 194–5

gauchos 138
gay fashion 118
ghetto blasters 181
Gina Shoes 94
girdles 21
glam rock 9, 151, 158
gloves 39, 43, 49–50, 75, 91
golf wear 27, 46, 97
Great Depression 15, 35
'greige' 144
'grunge' 187

hairstyles 113
  afro hair 131, 183
  beehives 131
  big hair 183
  bobs 131, 193
  chignons 101
  fringes 159

front quiff ponytails 101
  men's 30, 51, 77, 101, 130, 159, 183, 193, 195
  No.1 159
  punk 137
  The Rachel 193
  tousled 159
  women's 28, 31, 77, 101, 130–1, 159, 183, 192, 195
  zigzag partings 192
Halston 32, 33, 137, 147
hangers 198, 207
hats 28, 32–3, 43, 49–50, 75–6, 98
  bowler 28, 39, 87
  caps 28, 49
  cleaning 32
  cloche 28, 32
  fedora 49, 75, 77, 98
  groom's 106–11
  linings 32
  pill-box 32, 75
  restoration 32–3
  storage 33
  summer 157
  top 22, 23
  trilby 28, 49, 61, 98
head scarves 98
Hindmarch, Anya 194–5
Hip Hop 170
hippies 8–9, 119, 120, 136, 143, 156, 157
'Hiroshima chic' 169
Hollywood 21, 35, 39, 41, 64, 67, 93, 147
hot pants 146
housewives, perfect 81, 88

ice skating 47

jackets 59, 84, 86–7
  bolero 65

dinner 22, 43, 68, 170
  leather 73, 87, 169
  men's suit 18, 39, 69, 93
  Nehru 121
Jagger, Bianca 148
Japanese fashions 169
jewellery 29, 157
  chokers 191
  costume 49, 74, 99, 128–9, 180, 199
  gold 180
  simulated gemstones 49
Jordan, Michael 178
jump suits 141

kaftans 109, 137, 148
kimonos 20, 146
Klein, Calvin 139
knitwear
  Fair Isle 19
  leg warmers 179
  men's 19, 26, 46, 63, 85, 139, 145
  skinny ribs 139
  tennis 26
  twinsets 82
  women's 36, 46, 58, 82, 139, 145, 165, 201

lace 90
'Land Girls' 57
Lanvin, Jeanne 20, 41
Lauren, Ralph 142, 154
Laurent, Yves Saint 89, 116, 136, 145, 148
leather 73, 87, 169, 197
leg warmers 179
leotards 178
Liberty Arts fabrics 187
Lonsdale 126, 127
Louboutin, Christian 194–5

Mackintoshes 38

Madonna 82, 181
'Make Do and Mend' 8, 55, 74, 76, 211
make-up 31, 51, 65, 77, 100, 103, 113, 132–3, 158, 182, 192–3
man-made fibres 37
McCartney, Stella 185, 194
McQueen, Alexander 194
Miami Vice (TV Show) 170
'Mod' look 120, 125
Moschino Cheap & Chic 189
Moss, Kate 185
motor racing style 155
MTV 161

nail art 195
nautical themes 140
New Balance 127, 155
New Romantics 10, 175, 176
New York aesthetic 139
Nike 177, 178
Nutter, Tommy 120
nylon 37, 89

odours 198, 207
Olympic Games 72, 73
opera 23
overcoats 60–1, 92

Pan's People 149
patchwork 139
perfume 132–3
Petri, Ray 168
petticoats, repairing 208–9
pleats 65, 83, 85
Poiret, Paul 20
polyester 206
polyvinyl chloride (PVC) 116, 125
Pompadour 101

222

ponchos 138
'preppy' look 85, 97, 176
psychedelica 123
Pucci, Emilio 123, 129
Puma 154
punks 118, 137–8, 156–8, 175, 183

Quant, Mary 114, 115, 122, 131
quilting 139

rationing 55–9, 66
'rave scene' 161, 174, 190
rayon 27, 37, 41, 206
Red or Dead 11, 174, 190
repairing garments 208–9, 212–13
Rockers 113
roller-skating 155
'rude boy' style 118, 159, 168

sandals 153, 159
scarves 75, 98
Schiaparelli, Elsa 17, 20–1, 40, 147
separates 57, 59, 81, 149
Sex and the City (TV show) 191
SEX shop (Westwood) 138
shirts 43, 151, 187
    see also Vintage Weddings
shoddy yards 11
shoe clips 25
shoes 24–5
    ankle straps 124
    ballet pumps 94
    brogues 45, 95
    buying 199
    cork 44
    court 177
    creepers 95

deep-ridged sole 190
espadrilles 190
jelly 176
loafer slip-on 176
Mary Janes 24, 104
men's 25, 39, 44–5, 71, 95, 106–11, 125, 153, 176–7, 190
men's high heels 153
platforms 44, 152–3, 159
slingbacks 124
slip-on 95
spectator 45
sports 26, 127, 154–5
stilettos 94, 152
trainers (sneakers) 154, 155, 177
wedding 106–11
wedges 153, 159
women's 24–5, 44–5, 70–1, 94, 106–11, 124–5, 152–3, 176–7, 190
shorts 141, 146
shoulder pads 58, 77, 166, 173
silk 148, 206
Simpson, Wallis 35
sizing 13, 30, 197
ski wear 46–7, 97
skins, exotic 45
    see also fur
skirts
    hobble 83
    letting out 211
    mini 115
    pleated 83
    puffball 164
    rah-rah 164
'smart-casual' look 84, 190
Smith, Paul 187, 195
space travel 113, 114
sportswear 26–7, 46–7, 72–3, 96–7, 126–7,

154–5, 178–9
stain removal 207
stockings 21, 99, 100
suits 18–19, 38–9, 175
    demob 61
    double-breasted 19, 150
    five-button 121
    grooms 106–11
    Italian 93, 120
    lounge 38–9
    plus four 38–9
    power 163
    reefer 38–9
    safari 145
    single-breasted 19, 87, 120, 171
    tuxedos 93, 148, 150, 175
    unisex 190
    women's 163, 190
    Zoot suits 69
sunglasses 100, 128, 156
Swatch watches 181
'sweater girls' 36, 82
swimwear 27, 96

T-shirts 138, 166–7, 171, 186
tailoring 18–19, 39
tank tops 85, 139
tattoos 149, 195
Teddy Boys 79, 86, 93, 95, 101, 150
teens 70, 79, 96
tennis wear 26, 47, 72, 97, 179
ties 39, 43, 62, 107–11
    bow 68, 150
    kipper 151
tights 115, 183
top hat and tails 22, 23
topless models 138
tracksuits 126, 179
trims 37

trousers 17, 18, 43, 59, 85, 86, 121
    Capri pants 80
    loons 121
    pleated 85
    suit 39, 69, 87, 171
turbans 75, 156
tuxedos 93, 148, 150, 175
TV 161, 191
Twiggy 8, 113, 114
twinsets 82

Umbro 127
underwear 196
    men's 99, 143, 196
    women's 82, 196
unisex clothing 118, 125, 144–5, 167, 190
upcycling 13, 31, 139
utility clothing 55, 56, 63

Valentino 122
velvet 41, 207
Von Furstenberg, Diane 149

waifs 185
waistcoats 22, 39, 43, 63, 109–10, 150
waistlines 17
waists
    cinched 64, 67, 80, 91
    nipped 58
watches 48, 50, 181
weddings 102–11
Westwood, Vivienne 10, 53, 138, 165, 169, 183
wool 206
World War II 55–7, 61–2, 64

Y-fronts 143

zips, replacement 212–13

A DAVID & CHARLES BOOK
© F&W Media International, Ltd 2015

David & Charles is an imprint of F&W Media International, Ltd
Brunel House, Forde Close, Newton Abbot, TQ12 4PU, UK

F&W Media International, Ltd is a subsidiary of F+W Media, Inc
10151 Carver Road, Suite #200, Blue Ash, OH 45242, USA

Text © Wayne and Gerardine Hemingway 2015
Layout © F&W Media International, Ltd 2015

First published in the UK and USA in 2015

A catalogue record for this book is available from the British Library.

ISBN-13: 978-1-4463-0441-9 hardback
ISBN-10: 1-4463-0441-8 hardback

ISBN-13: 978-1-4463-6576-2 PDF
ISBN-10: 1-4463-6576-X PDF

Printed in China by RR Donnelley for:
F&W Media International, Ltd
Brunel House, Forde Close, Newton Abbot, TQ12 4PU, UK

10 9 8 7 6 5 4 3 2 1

Managing Editor: Honor Head
Creative Director: Rita Lopes
Copy Editor: Jean Coppendale
Designer: Emma Wicks
Picture research: Hannah Wing, Jean Coppendale
Production Manager: Beverley Richardson

F+W Media publishes high quality books on a wide range of subjects.
For more great book ideas visit: **www.stitchcraftcreate.co.uk**

Layout of the digital edition of this book may vary depending on reader hardware and display settings.

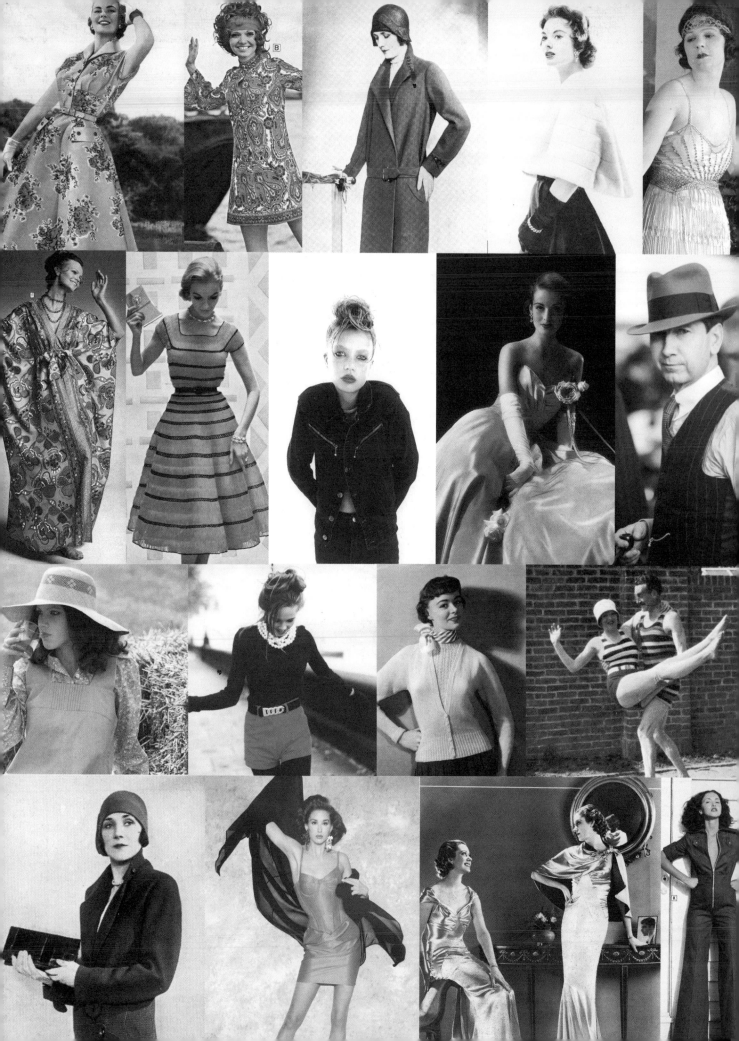